CONTENTS

CHURCHILL'S POCKETBOOK OF
Intensive Care

For Churchill Livingstone:

Publisher: Michael Parkinson
Project Editor: Janice Urquhart
Copy Editor: Therese Duriez
Indexer: Monica Trigg
Design Direction: Erik Bigland
Project Controller: Kay Hunston

UK: Freephone 0500 566 242
Europe: + 44 131 535 1021
USA/Canada: + 1 201 319 9800
Australia/New Zealand: + 61 3 9699 5400

CHURCHILL'S POCKETBOOK OF
Intensive Care

Simon M. Whiteley

MB BS FRCA
Consultant, Intensive Care,
The General Infirmary at Leeds
Leeds, UK

Andrew Bodenham

MB BS FRCA
Consultant, Intensive Care,
The General Infirmary at Leeds, Leeds, UK

Mark C. Bellamy

MA MB BS FRCA
Consultant, Intensive Care,
St James's University Hospital, Leeds, UK

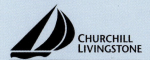

CHURCHILL
LIVINGSTONE

EDINBURGH LONDON NEW YORK PHILADELPHIA
SAN FRANCISCO SYDNEY TORONTO 1998

CHURCHILL LIVINGSTONE
A Division of Harcourt Brace and Company Limited

Robert Stevenson House, 1—3 Baxter's Place,
Leith Walk, Edinburgh EH1 3AF, UK

First published 1998

ISBN 0 443 0 5363 4

British Library of Cataloguing in Publication Data
A catalogue record for this book is available from the
British Library.

Library of Congress Cataloging in Publication Data
A catalog record for this book is available from the
Library of Congress.

Illustrated by David Gardner

Medical knowledge is constantly changing. As new
information becomes available, changes in treatment,
procedures, equipment and the use of drugs become
necessary. The authors and the publishers have, as far
as it is possible, taken care to ensure that the
information given in this text is accurate and up to
date. However, readers are strongly advised to
confirm that the information, especially with regard
to drug usage, complies with current legislation and
standards of practice.

Printed in Singapore

Preface

This small book follows other successful titles in the Churchill's pocketbook format. It is not intended to compete with the many already well-established texts in the field of intensive care, but is intended to present a distillation of sensible practice and ideas.

Every new doctor who is resident in the intensive care unit will be faced by a large variety of clinical problems to be solved. This book is therefore based on the common problems the authors are asked about on a regular basis, most of which can be easily solved by following simple rules. The aim has been to use the minimum of space, by avoiding excessive detail, and no apology is made for repetition, or for what may on occasion appear a didactic approach. Information related to the specialist areas such as paediatric and cardiothoracic intensive care has been specifically excluded, although the general principles described are equally applicable in these areas.

In many countries there are increasing moves to rotate trainees from different specialties, without previous intensive care experience, through intensive care. The hope is that this guide will prove timely and useful in this respect.

S. M. W.   1998
A. B.
M. C. B.

Contents

Abbreviations

A&E	accident and emergency
ACE	angiotensin converting enzyme
ACN	acute cortical necrosis
ADH	antidiuretic hormone
AF	atrial fibrillation
AIDS	acquired immune deficiency syndrome
ANA	antinuclear antibodies
ANCA	antineutrophil cytoplasmic antibodies
APTT	activated partial thromboplastin time
ARDS	acute respiratory distress syndrome
ARF	acute renal failure
ASB	assisted spontaneous breathing
AST	aspartate aminotransferase
ATLS	advanced trauma life support
ATN	acute tubular necrosis
AV	arteriovenous
BAL	bronchial alveolar lavage
BMR	basal metabolic rate
BNF	British National Formulary
BP	blood pressure
BSA	body surface area
CCU	coronary care unit
CFM	cerebral function monitor
CK	creatinine kinase
CMV	cytomegalovirus
CMV	controlled mandatory ventilation
CNS	central nervous system
COAD	chronic obstructive airways disease
CO	cardiac output
CPAP	continuous positive airway pressure
CPP	cerebral perfusion pressure
CRF	chronic renal failure
CSF	cerebrospinal fluid
CSSD	central sterile supplies department
CT	computerized tomography
CVP	central venous pressure
CXR	chest X-ray
DDAVP	desmopressin
DI	diabetes insipidus
DIC	disseminated intravascular coagulation
DKA	diabetic ketoacidosis
DVT	deep venous thrombosis
EBV	Epstein-Barr virus
ECF	extra cellular fluid
ECG	electrocardiogram
FBC	full blood count
FDP	fibrin degradation product
FFP	fresh frozen plasma
FRC	functional residual capacity
GCS	Glasgow coma scale
GCSF	granulocyte-colony stimulating factor
GFR	glomerular filtration rate
GIT	gastrointestinal tract
GTN	glyceryl trinitrate
GU	genitourinary

HDU	high dependency unit	**PEEP**	positive end expiratory pressure
HELLP	haemolysis, elevated liver enzymes, low platelets	**PEG**	percutaneous endoscopic gastrostomy
HIV	human immunodeficiency virus	**PPV**	positive pressure ventilation
		PT	prothrombin time
ICP	intracranial pressure		
ICU	intensive care unit	**RAST**	radioallergosorbant tests
IPPV	intermittent positive pressure ventilation	**RV**	right ventricle
ISS	injury severity score	**SAG-M**	saline-adenine-glucose with mannitol
IU	international unit	**SAH**	subarachnoid haemorrhage
IVP	intravenous pyelogram	**SCID**	severe combined immune deficiency
		SDD	selective decontamination digestive tract
LP	lumbar puncture		
LDH	lactate dehydrogenase	**SIADH**	syndrome of inappropriate antidiuretic hormone
LVEDV	left ventricular end diastolic volume	**SIMV**	synchronized intermittent mandatory ventilation
MAP	mean arterial pressure	**SIRS**	systemic inflammatory response syndrome
MABP	mean arterial blood pressure	**SLE**	systemic lupus erythematosus
MH	malignant hyperpyrexia	**SVR**	systemic vascular resistance
MOF	multiple organ failure		
MRSA	methicillin resistant staphylococcus aureus	**SVT**	supraventricular tachycardia
NMR	nuclear magnetic resonance	**TCD**	transcranial doppler
NSAIDs	non-steroidal anti-inflammatory drugs	**TEG**	thromboelastogram
		TNF	tumour necrosis factor
REM	rapid eye movement	**TPN**	total parenteral nutrition
		TSH	thyroid stimulating hormone
PA	pulmonary artery	**TT**	thrombin time
PAF	platelet activating factor		
PAFC	pulmonary artery flotation catheter	**VPB**	ventricular premature beat
PAOP	pulmonary artery occlusion pressure	**VSD**	ventricular septal defect
		VT	ventricular tachycardia
PCAS	patient controlled analgesic system	**WBC**	white blood cell
PCP	pneumocystis carinii pneumonia	**WCC**	white cell count
PCR	polymerase chain reaction		

INTRODUCTION

AIMS AND DEFINITIONS

Intensive care fulfils a number of roles. These include:

- Physiological optimization of patients to prevent the onset of organ failure.
- Facilitation of complex surgery.
- Support of failing organ systems.

What constitutes an Intensive Care Unit (ICU) is open to debate but there are useful definitions which try to separate the function of intensive care and high dependency care.

Intensive care

Intensive care is an area for patients admitted for the treatment of actual or impending organ failure especially those requiring assisted ventilation. There is usually one nurse per patient throughout the day and a doctor assigned solely to the intensive care throughout the 24-hour period.

Intensive care is very expensive. Typical UK costs are around £1500 per day. The larger part of this expenditure relates to staffing costs, drugs and disposables. For example in the larger units typical nursing numbers are 6–8 whole time equivalents per staffed bed space. In the UK approximately 1% of hospital beds are intensive care beds, whereas in the USA the comparable figure is 10%.

In the early days of intensive care patients were often young, previously fit, with single organ failure and full recovery could be expected. Today, patients are increasingly elderly, with extensive pre-existing medical problems, and often present with multiple organ failure. The realization of the large costs involved in treating patients with limited prospect for survival, has resulted in the value of intensive care being questioned.

High dependency care

High dependency is an area for patients who require more intensive observation and interventions than can be performed on a general ward. This would normally exclude patients requiring assisted ventilation. Nursing levels are generally between those of an ICU and a general ward. There is not usually dedicated medical cover.

There are difficulties with such definitions. In many smaller hospitals, ICU, High Dependency Units (HDUs) and Coronary Care Units (CCUs) are often combined in one area with flexible working of nursing and medical staff to cover clinical needs on a day-to-day basis. Whatever the practicality of local arrangements, the concept of staged care, where sick patients move from intensive care to high dependency care and then to the general ward care, is increasingly practicable.

MULTIDISCIPLINARY APPROACH

The care of patients in intensive care is increasingly complex, and the specialization of medical staff precludes all care being provided by a single individual or team. The critically ill patient is cared for in a central area, where he/she receives optimum care and input from a number of different specialities. A major role for junior and senior medical staff in intensive care is the coordination of all aspects of patient care, and in particular the maintenance of good lines of communication between the different teams involved.

There are many other nursing, paramedical and technical staff involved in the care of patients on intensive care. It is important to remember that all these people have skills and experience that you do not. Do not be afraid to ask for advice. If you treat them as colleagues you will get more from them. In particular those listed below should be consulted.

Nursing staff

Many nursing staff in the ICU are very experienced and very knowledgeable. You should see them as allies and listen to and carefully consider their advice. Remember also that nurses have their own job to do which is demanding and time consuming. They are not there to run about after you. Therefore if you can get something you need – get it, and clear up your own mess after you!

Physiotherapists

Physiotherapists provide therapy for clearance of chest secretions. They have an important role in helping to maintain joint and limb function in bed-bound patients, and in mobilizing patients during their recovery. They can often provide help with the respiratory care and management of patients on the general wards who are struggling to maintain adequate respiratory function and who might otherwise require admission to intensive care. You should listen to their advice.

Pharmacists

The nature of intensive care is such that patients will often be on many medications. There is, therefore, a great potential for drug interactions and incompatibility of infusions. In addition many drug doses need modification in the presence of hepatic and renal failure. The pharmacist will generally review prescriptions and is a ready source of advice on all therapeutic matters.

Dieticians

All patients in intensive care require some form of nutrition. While basic nutritional support can be provided by standard regimens, many hospitals now have nutrition teams including dieticians who will tailor regimens to each patient's particular requirements.

Technicians

There are a large number of technical staff involved in supporting the ICU. These include laboratory technicians, renal technicians who manage haemodialysis machines, and equipment service engineers. Cultivate a good relationship with all these people. They can be an invaluable source of help.

ADMISSION POLICIES

The aim of intensive care is to support patients while they recover. It is not to prolong life when there is no hope of recovery. Sometimes difficult decisions have to be made about whether or not to admit a patient to intensive care, particularly since there is a general shortage of intensive care beds and a requirement to use the available resources responsibly. To aid such decisions some units have written admission policies. For example:

Admission policy

Requests for admission

- Will come from a consultant who has seen the patient immediately prior to admission.
- Will be made by contacting the consultant on-call for intensive care.
- In the case of elective surgery where the admission of the patient can be foreseen a request should be made at least 24 hours prior to surgery. The bed should be confirmed immediately prior to surgery.

Admission policy

- All problems related to availability of beds will be dealt with initially by the ICU consultant on-call who is in a position to make decisions about the potential admission and the needs of the patients already in the ICU.
- If the ICU is full it may be possible to transfer a patient out to free a bed; if this is not possible provision of care at an appropriate level will remain the responsibility of the consultant who is in charge of the case.
- The ICU consultant may give advice as to which local ICU may have room but the prime responsibility of the consultant is to provide care for the patients in the ICU.
- Determining which patients are suitable for intensive care when there are insufficient beds is a complex issue that can only be determined by a doctor with knowledge of all the relevant cases. Patients already undergoing treatment in the ICU will be given priority over a potential admission. There are circumstances where transfer of a current patient to another ICU may be appropriate if a potential admission is undergoing a course of therapy that cannot be provided at another local hospital.

Joint responsibility

● All patients will be under the care of an intensive care consultant but usually ultimate responsibility will remain with the consultant from the admitting team.
● Continuity of care through critical illness will be provided by the intensive care junior and senior staff. In the interests of continuity it remains the responsibility of the non- ICU doctors to communicate any change in therapy with the ICU team.

Discharges

● Will be arranged by the ICU staff in conjunction with responsible consultant. In cases of emergency, however, patients may be discharged by the consultant on-call for the ICU.

The difficulty with all admission policies is that it is impossible to predict with accuracy which individual patients stand to benefit from admission to intensive care. On this basis, patients are often admitted for a trial of therapy to see whether they will stabilize and improve over time.

Inevitably, on occasion, truly hopeless cases will be admitted. For example, patients from the resuscitation room, or those who have suffered catastrophic complications during surgery, may be admitted even though they are likely to die. This allows the relatives time to visit and the bereavement process to be better managed. Medicolegal considerations may also be relevant in this context. Admission policies should therefore be flexible enough to allow admission of what may seem like a hopeless case.

PREDICTION OF OUTCOME

The difficulties outlined above have led to a wealth of work, using scoring systems to predict outcome of patients treated in intensive care. This generally involves the collection of a large amount of data from many patients, stratification of the data to produce a risk score, and then the application of the risk score to individuals. There are major difficulties however with this approach:

● There is as yet, no satisfactory diagnostic categorization for intensive care patients. Often the problems relating to intensive care admission bear little relation to the original presenting complaint or diagnostic category.
● Although patients may survive to leave the ICU there is a significant mortality on the wards and later at home after leaving intensive care. Many studies use 28-day mortality as an end point. It is argued that 6 month/ 1 year outcomes of mortality and measures of morbidity (quality of life measures) are better end points.

● Scoring systems which attempt to quantify degree of sickness have proved unreliable for prediction in individual cases. The best known of these is the APACHE score. A high APACHE score which takes in to account both acute physiological disturbances and the chronic health of the patient correlates well with the risk of death for the intensive care population as a whole. This score has been used with computer modelling to predict outcome for an individual, (e.g. Riyadh Intensive Care Programme) but this approach has tended to generate adverse publicity.

In practice most units use simple clinical decision making to decide which patients to admit to the ICU. In many cases unless the outlook is truly hopeless patients will be admitted for a trial of treatment. Instantaneous judgements regarding continuation or withdrawal of treatment in patients in the operating theatre, resuscitation room or on the wards, are potentially dangerous. Critics will point out that decisions to discontinue treatment on grounds of futility become self-fulfilling prophecies. Senior staff should be involved from the outset. (See APACHE scoring, p. 40.)

DISCHARGE POLICIES

Generally because of the pressure on intensive care beds, discharge policies are just as hard to define as admission policies. Patients may be discharged in the following circumstances.

● The patient's condition has improved to the extent that intensive care is no longer required and is therefore inappropriate.
● The patient's condition is not improving and the underlying problems are such that continued intensive care is futile In such cases it is imperative that the general ward staff, the patient's family and where possible the patient, agree that such decisions are appropriate and that the decision is clearly documented.

For patients whose condition is improving and for whom discharge is considered, two questions have to be asked:

I. When are patients fit to be discharged?
In simple terms patients are fit for discharge from intensive care when they no longer require the specialist skills and monitoring available on the intensive care unit. This generally means that they have no life threatening organ failure and that their underlying disease process is stable or improving. Table 1.1 gives some guidance.

TABLE 1.1 Criteria for discharge	
Airway	Adequate airway & cough to clear secretions (Alternatively tracheostomy and suction)
Breathing	Adequate respiratory effort and blood gases. Not needing respiratory support. May be oxygen dependant from mask

Circulation	Cardiovascularly stable
	Not on any inotropes
Neurological function	Adequate conscious level
	Adequate cough and gag reflexes as above
	If bulbar palsy or brain injury may need tracheostomy to make
	airway safe and allow airway toilet
Renal function	Adequate renal function and urine output
	(Unless discharged to renal unit)
	May be on renal dose dopamine
Analgesia	Adequate simple analgesia

2. Where is the patient to be sent?

This will depend at least in part on the patient's underlying diagnosis, current condition, and where the patient came from in the first place. Some patients, especially elective postoperative surgical patients, may be fit enough to go straight back to a general ward. Others may, because of continuing organ dysfunction or other problems, require closer monitoring, supervision and nursing care and may go back to an HDU.

Occasionally patients who have been transferred from another ICU for specialist treatment or because of lack of beds may be discharged back to the referring hospital. In general patients should be returned to their referring hospital as soon as possible, if only for the sake of relatives who may find travelling difficult. This may require a medical escort.
(See Transporting patients, p. 266.)

Communication

Whenever a patient is transferred out of intensive care, whether to high dependency care, a general ward, or another hospital, you should inform the referring medical staff. You should provide a brief written summary of the patient's intensive care treatment together with a guide to ongoing airway, respiratory and cardiovascular management.

It is always wise to let the patient's family know that transfers are to take place. Relatives and patients quickly become used to and come to expect, the level of care received in the ICU, and often complain about care on the general wards as a result. Moves to the ward need to be placed in a positive light as a step forward for the patient. HDUs provide an invaluable step-down facility in this respect.

TALKING TO RELATIVES

The relatives of critically ill patients may well ask to speak to a doctor about the patient's condition or you may request to speak to them. Discussions with relatives should generally take place in a quiet room away from the patient's beside.

● Do not talk over the patient; they may be aware of their surroundings and able to hear. (Hearing is the last sensory modality to be lost with sedative drugs.)

● Do not talk standing in the corridor; use a side room away from other families.

● It is always advisable to take a nurse with you so that he or she knows what has been said. The relatives will probably only retain a fraction of what has been said to them, and the nurse can reinforce what you have said later. The nurse may also offer comfort and moral support to the patient's family.

● Adjust the explanation of events to the level of intelligence/experience of the relatives and avoid medical jargon and abbreviations.

● It is always sensible to be as honest as possible with relatives and not to be over-optimistic about the ability of intensive care to turn around desperate situations. There are inherent uncertainties about the outcome of any particular disease and it is best to be cautious rather than giving 'exact' probabilities of survival.

● Do not criticize medical or nursing colleagues' management of the patient. It is all too easy, with the benefit of hindsight, to see where things went wrong, but you may have done no better yourself on the wards without all the facilities and expertise available to the ICU. Difficult questions or decisions should be referred upwards to the consultant in charge.

● Do not let family members push you into making statements that are not true. This is particularly important concerning prognosis. Don't agree with statements like 'He is going to be all right isn't he Doctor' if it is not true.

● In the medical notes record in simple terms what has been said to the family. This ensures continuity and prevents misunderstandings.

(See Confidentiality, p. 11 and Breaking bad news, p. 14.)

ETHICAL AND LEGAL ISSUES

The ethical and legal aspects of intensive care are still a matter for debate. Acceptable medical practice changes subtly with time whilst the confirmed legal opinion may lag behind. Advances in the technology and practice of intensive care medicine have enabled patients to be kept alive with little hope of recovery. Decisions to limit or withdraw therapy then have to be made. These decisions are always difficult, and will occasionally result in differences of opinion between both professionals and patients and their families. Therefore try to see issues from other people's perspectives.

 Warning! Always seek help regarding more difficult ethical and legal decisions such as withdrawal of therapy.

MEDICAL NOTES

Intensive care is a multidisciplinary speciality, and many different doctors may be involved in the care of a patient. The patient's condition may also change rapidly requiring frequent changes in therapy. Therefore if everyone is to keep up with the patient's progress, accurate, contemporaneous note keeping is essential. You should record:

- Daily examination and progress notes.
- Interventions and procedures
- Complications of procedures must be recorded accurately and honestly. Complications do occur and providing you have followed correct procedures, complications do not imply negligence. (Failure to record them or act appropriately upon them does!)
- Results of important investigations.
- The patient's chart is often used to record blood gases, biochemistry, haematology and microbiology results. This is a legal document and therefore the results do not need to be routinely copied into the medical notes. Important positive and negative findings however, particularly those which carry either diagnostic or prognostic significance or which directly affect management should be transcribed.
- It is useful to record the content and outcome of discussion with the patient's relatives, so that other staff do not give conflicting advice or opinions.

Occasionally because of the pressure of work in the ICU it may not be possible to make full notes at the time, for example when admitting and resuscitating a very unstable patient. It is crucial however, that notes are written at the earliest opportunity and the fact that they have been written retrospectively, recorded.

CONSENT TO TREATMENT

Consent is a difficult area in intensive care. Except for elective admissions after major surgery patients will often have had no opportunity to discuss intensive care treatment before admission. They are admitted to ICUs on the presumption that they would wish to undergo life sustaining treatments, if given the choice. The validity of obtaining consent from third parties (e.g. spouses, partners, other relatives, etc.) is questionable in this context. Nevertheless, it is considered normal practice to do so, and relatives expect it.

When is written consent required?

Patients in the ICU will have repeated interventions performed, for example, tracheal suction, arterial and venous line insertion, and passage of tubes into various orifices. Most units would not seek specific consent for these procedures, but you should always explain to the patient, and their relatives if present, what you are going to do.

For more significant invasive procedures like returning to theatre for re-laparotomy, tracheostomy, insertion of intracranial pressure monitoring, it is usual to seek consent whenever possible.

Patients requiring intensive care are, however, usually unfit to give consent. Despite theoretical invalidity of informed consent from relatives, it is usually good practice to inform them that such procedures are to take place and inform them of the likely risks. Most hospital consent forms have a section for third party consent and it is usual practice to obtain it. If the relatives are not present then it is courteous and avoids conflict to obtain consent over the telephone. If nothing else, it ensures relatives are kept informed and provides an opportunity for an update on the patient's condition. Relatives do not respond well to news of the death of a patient in the operating theatre, when they did not know that an operation was planned, and time would have allowed for a telephone call!

It is unusual for relatives to refuse consent, but it may occur on occasions, in which case the medical staff are left with the difficult decision whether to carry on against the relatives' wishes or not. With an adult it can be argued that relatives have no right to intervene. In a child under the legal age of consent (16 years) application may be made for the child to be made a ward of court, and the court's consent to treatment obtained. If there is any difficulty with consent seek senior help.

There is an increasing number of specific circumstances where one might expect to be refused consent.

Jehovah's Witnesses

Jehovah's Witnesses have religious objections to receiving transfusions of blood or blood products. Where these views are declared it is usual practice to discuss with the patient what therapy they will and will not accept, and then to obtain a written disclaimer from the patient. They should then be managed in the appropriate way but *without* the use of blood products. The situation in intensive care is difficult if the patient is unable to express his/her view at the time; if there is sufficient evidence of the patient's religious beliefs, these should be respected.

The situation with children is different. The child should be brought under the protection of the courts and a life saving blood transfusion should be given. (See Blood transfusion, p. 154 and management of Jehovah's Witnesses, p. 157.)

Advance directives

An increasing number of people are writing so-called Advance Directives to outline what treatment they would or would not wish to have performed in the future in the case of them being unfit to make this decision at the time. The best known scenarios for such directives come from patients who are human immunodeficiency virus (HIV) positive with acquired immune deficiency syndrome (AIDS) and patients with progressive dementia. In the case of HIV patients the directive may take the form of a request that they are not admitted to intensive care for assisted ventilation in the case of severe opportunistic pneumonia. At the time of writing, the exact legal status of such documents in the UK is still under discussion. It seems reasonable however, that such decisions if properly set out should be respected. This may make the doctor's role in clinical decision making very much easier.

Organ donor cards

People are encouraged to outline their wishes regarding potential organ donation by carrying signed organ donor cards and registering on the national data base. This could be considered a form of advance directive. (See Brain-stem death, p. 181 and organ donation, p. 184.)

HIV TESTING

The ethical guidelines on HIV testing are clear. Patients cannot be tested for HIV infection without informed consent, which is taken to include adequate counselling both before the test and after a positive test result. The situation in intensive care therefore is difficult, since it is unlikely that informed consent can be obtained.

As an HIV test does not often alter the management of, for example, a severe opportunistic infection, HIV tests should not be performed until the patient is over his/her acute illness and adequate informed consent can be obtained. In particular:

● You cannot perform an HIV test for the benefit of staff who consider that they may be at risk from blood contamination, etc. Universal precautions should be adopted with all patients to avoid occupational risk.
● The decision to perform an HIV test should be made by a consultant.

CONFIDENTIALITY

The patient's medical condition and treatment, is a matter of confidentiality. While it is generally accepted in intensive care that relatives should be kept informed of what is going on you must respect the patient's wishes and confidentiality at all times. Therefore:

● Make sure you know to whom you are talking before giving out any information.
● Never discuss a patient's condition on the telephone. You do not know who is on the other end of the line. The press have been known to telephone and not admit who they are. If a relative lives too far away to make it to the hospital, offer to telephone them back on a previously agreed number.
● Never make any comment to journalists. Refer them to your hospital press liaison officer or your consultant.

● Occasionally the police may request information about a patient or request a blood test. The same rules apply no matter what the patient may have done. If in doubt refer them to your consultant.

DEALING WITH DEATH

In an average larger ICU there is a 15–25% on-unit mortality. In addition significant numbers of patients die soon after discharge from ITU. Therefore dealing with death and the ethical and legal issues surrounding it are very important. If death is handled sympathetically and with dignity relatives will generally be grateful and any minor complaints they may have had are often forgotten!

With most patients who die on intensive care, decisions are made that active treatment should be either withdrawn, reduced or not increased. Such decisions are more common than 'do not resuscitate' orders as practised on general wards.

Withdrawal of treatment

Commonly patients will be admitted to the ICU for a period of stabilization and assessment. Over time, however, it becomes clear that the prognosis is hopeless and that the patient has no prospect of useful recovery. It is in such patients that decisions are made regarding withdrawal of treatment.

● There is no medicolegal obligation to carry on treatment when it is futile.
● There should be a consensus from all clinicians and nursing staff involved with care of the patient that continuation of active management is inappropriate.

While there is no requirement to obtain consent from family members or relatives regarding withdrawal of treatment, it is good clinical practice to involve the family as far as possible and to be honest. Most relatives appreciate time spent in explanation and will accept the concept of withdrawal of treatment. Discussion with relatives should be led by an appropriate consultant, either from the referring team or from the ICU.

The best practice in terms of withdrawing treatment is open to debate. From a legal point of view there is no distinction drawn between, for example, the withdrawal of vasoactive drugs and assisted ventilation. Normally drug therapy and ventilation would be reduced slowly to minimize distress to the patient. Maintenance fluids and nutrition are continued to aid patient comfort.

Warning! The withdrawal of life sustaining therapy such as nasogastric feeding from patients in Persistent Vegetative State, who otherwise do not require any form of organ support is a complex legal issue. This would normally take place outside the ICU and is beyond the scope of this book.

Euthanasia

UK law does not allow the practice of euthanasia. Patients who are dying should not, however, be allowed to suffer needlessly. It is permissible to administer sedative or analgesic drugs to relieve patient distress, accepting that in some cases the administration of these drugs will speed up the process of death. Most units would prescribe benzodiazepines or opiates for this purpose and many relatives gain comfort from the fact that the dying patient is not allowed to suffer.

Managing death

Consideration should be given as to where is the best place for a patient to die. The process is usually best managed in intensive care, where the patient and relatives can be supported by the staff. Some units are now developing so-called 'tender loving care' rooms specifically designed for this purpose. If the patient's bed is likely to be required in the near future it may be appropriate to transfer the patient to a general ward. Consideration should also be given to the timing of withdrawal of therapy in order that relatives visiting from afar may be present.

Relatives often ask how long death will take but this can be very difficult to predict. Some patients may survive a few minutes, others a few hours. Occasionally a patient may even apparently improve temporarily following withdrawal of inotropes. Therefore, be honest and say that you do not know!

Confirming death

When a patient dies, death must be confirmed by a doctor. Generally note:

- Absence of palpable pulse. Absence of heart sounds.
- Absence of respiratory effort (disconnect ventilator).
- Pupils are fixed and dilated.

Write these observations, with the date and exact time of death in the notes and sign them.

 Warning! Confirming death in severely hypothermic patients is very difficult. In general patients cannot be dead until they are warm and dead. This may require heroic attempts at resuscitation and rewarming for example in victims of cold water immersion. In doubt seek help (See Hypothermia, p. 146.)

Whom to inform

Once death is confirmed you must make sure that the relatives have been informed (see below). You should also inform the people listed below although this can often wait until the next morning if the patient has died out of hours. Actions will depend upon the circumstances and in, particular, whether the death was expected or not.

- Referring clinician(s).
- Consultant in charge of intensive care.
- The patient's general practitioner. (This is especially important. It fosters good relations between the hospital and the community and allows the GP an opportunity to offer counselling and support to the relatives.)
- Coroner's officer if appropriate (see below).

Breaking bad news

This is never an easy task, particularly if the death has occurred unexpectedly or if the patient was very young. If the relatives are not present at the time of the death they will generally be called by a senior nurse and asked to come into the hospital. Try to avoid talking on the telephone if at all possible. When they are present or when they arrive you should speak to them in a quiet side room. It is worth checking that all relevant members of the family are present since different branches of families may not communicate.

- Follow the basic guide above on talking to relatives.
- You must be honest but not brutal! Relatives may find it helpful to know that their loved one was not in any pain or distress.

The stages of bereavement include denial, anger and gradual acceptance. Any of these emotions may be expressed. It is not uncommon for a relative's initial response to take the form of anger if things have gone badly for his/her relative. Such anger will often subside over time as the realities of the situation become apparent. Sympathetic handling, honesty and compassion with relatives avoids many later complaints or medicolegal actions from patients' families.

   Many units now offer relatives the chance to return at a later date to revisit the sequence of events surrounding a patient's death and to ask any questions that they may still have. This is a valuable part of the grieving process for relatives.

ISSUING A DEATH CERTIFICATE

The death certificate asks you to give information about the cause of death. You can issue a death certificate if:

- You have been in attendance on the patient during his last illness, and you have seen the patient alive within 14 days of the death. (28 days in Scotland and Northern Ireland.)
- You are satisfied that the death was due to natural causes(see below).
- You are reasonably sure of the cause of death.

   If you can issue a death certificate, then complete the relevant sections. The death certificate is then given to the patient's family so that it can register the death. In many hospitals a bereavement liaison officer will handle these matters. Ensure that you fill in the form accurately, as it is very distressing for relatives if the certificate is rejected by the registrar.

Hospital postmortem examinations

Where the cause of death is known but information from a postmortem would be of interest you may ask the family for a hospital postmortem. Where a death occurs after major surgery, most surgeons will require a postmortem. This may help clarify the events leading up to the death. There is space on the death certificate to record that more information may be available from a postmortem subsequently.

Warning! If the cause of death is not clear then you must not ask for a hospital postmortem. In this instance the death must be reported to the coroner.

REPORTING DEATHS TO THE CORONER

If you are unable to issue a death certificate you must report the death to the coroner (procurator fiscal in Scotland). In addition there are a number of specific circumstances in which the death must be reported.

Indication for reporting death to the coroner

Death within 24 hours of hospital admission
Death occurring in the operating theatre
Death relating to surgery or anaesthesia*
Death due to accidents and trauma including assaults
Death associated with abortion spontaneous or induced
Death due to poisoning, or misuse of drugs
Death associated with neglect, including self-neglect
Death associated with industrial disease

*It is advisable to discuss any death following surgery with the coroner. There is no formal time limit laid down for this.

If in any doubt about what you should do, you should discuss the death with the coroner. You will generally deal with the coroner's officer. These are usually police appointments with variable degrees of medical knowledge but are nevertheless, a useful source of advice.

When speaking to the coroner's officer you will need the following information:

● Deceased patient's name, date of birth, address.
● Address and telephone number of next of kin and GP.
● Brief summary of the patient's last illness, including date of admission, diagnosis, operations, complications, and date and time of death.
● Reason for reporting death.
● Suggested cause of death if prepared to offer a death certificate.

If the cause of death is not suspicious, or unnatural the coroner may give permission for you to issue a death certificate (initial box 'A' on the reverse of the death certificate). In this case the cause of death cited on the form is agreed with the coroner's officer who then issues a covering slip to the registrar's office.

If the cause of death is unknown, or is suspicious or unnatural then the coroner's officer will take over. Generally a coroner's postmortem will be performed, and if necessary an inquest convened.

Situation in Scotland

In Scotland the situation is slightly different. The procurator fiscal investigates deaths reported to him/her. His/her main concern is to establish evidence of negligence or criminality rather than the cause of death. If satisfied that the death is natural the procurator fiscal may instruct a doctor to examine the body and issue a death certificate. If the cause of death is suspicious an application must be made to the sheriff for a postmortem examination. The cause of death is then certified by the pathologist. If there is evidence of negligence or criminality, then the lord advocate may order that a fatal accident enquiry be held.

BRAIN-STEM DEATH AND ORGAN DONATION

The brain stem is responsible for the maintenance of life sustaining functions within the body, in particular the maintenance and adequacy of respiration. With the advent of modern intensive care it is possible for patients in whom brain-stem death has occurred to be on a ventilator and still have a heart beat and pulse. These patients are not capable of sustaining life on their own. Therefore brain-stem death is now a legally accepted definition of death, the diagnosis of which is governed by strict guidelines and protocols. (See Brain–stem death p. 181.)

Patients who are brain-stem dead and on a ventilator may be suitable for organ donation. Although organ donor cards may be considered an advanced directive, it is good practice to discuss the issue of organ donation with the relatives and ask them for permission to remove organs from their relative. You may also need to ask permission of the coroner if the case would normally have been reported to the coroner. (*See above.*)

Note not all people will give consent to organ donation, some religious groups in particular find it difficult. You must accept their wishes no matter what your own views are. (See Organ donation, p. 184.)

DEATH AND DIFFERENT CULTURAL VIEWS

Different religious groups have different ways of dealing with death. This may clash with your own religious or cultural beliefs. Some groups may have large extended families and display 'exaggerated' grief. A number of religious groups are unhappy about postmortem examinations and some prefer to remove the body from the hospital as soon as possible after death. This can sometimes be arranged. You should try to respect the views of others.

Table 1.2 gives a brief guide to the beliefs and practices of the more common religious groups.

● Routine care of the dying and last offices are appropriate unless otherwise stated.
● There is no religious objection to postmortem examination or organ donation unless otherwise stated.

TABLE 1.2 Beliefs and practices of common religious groups	
Anglicans	May request Baptism, Eucharist, or Anointing.
Roman Catholics	May request Baptism, Holy Communion & Sacrament of the dying.
Free Church	Christians who do not conform to the Anglican or Catholic tradition. Generally less emphasis on the sacraments. May request a minister for informal prayers.
Jehovah's Witnesses	Unrestricted access family and friends and church elders. (There are no formal ministers, all Jehovah's Witnesses are ministers.) There are no ceremonial rites at death.
Christian Scientists	Believe in the power of God's healing and avoid conventional medicine. May accept conventional medicine due to family or legal pressure without loss of faith and allow medical care of children. No specific ceremonial rites at death. Would not wish to consent to postmortem or organ donation.
Afro-Caribbean Community	Extended family and church visits. More emphasis on prayer than sacraments. May prefer for body to be handled by staff of same cultural background. Older members of the community may believe in the sanctity of the body and not wish to consent to postmortem or organ donation.
Rastafarians	May prefer alternative therapy to conventional medicine. Distinctive hairstyle. Orthodox may not want hair cut. Second hand clothes are taboo, may be reluctant to wear hospital gowns. No specific ceremonial rites at death. Unlikely to consent to postmortem or organ donation.
Buddhists	State of mind is important. Require peace and quiet for meditation and chanting may help. May request counselling from local Buddhists. No specific ceremonial rites at death. A Buddhist monk should be informed of the death.

Jews	Orthodox Jews will wish to maintain customs of dress, diet, prayer and observe the Sabbath whilst in hospital.
	Object to any intervention which may hasten death (e.g. withdrawal of treatment) and families may wish to consult a rabbi.
	No specific ceremonial rites at death but may recite special prayers.
	There is a wish that dying Jews should not be left alone.
	Ritual laying out of the body by Jewish burial society with burial arranged ideally within 24 hours.
	Postmortem not permitted except where law requires it.
	Unlikely to consent to organ donation.
Muslims	Muslim women will not want to be seen by male doctors.
	Prayer rituals may be continued.
	Cleanliness important and running water required for washing.
	Friends and family may recite prayer, dying patient may wish to be turned towards Mecca (south-east).
	Body should not be touched by non-Muslims (if necessary wear gloves) and should be prepared according to the wishes of the family or priest.
	Funerals should take place within 24 hours where possible.
	Believe in the sanctity of the body.
	Unlikely to consent to postmortem or organ donation.
Hindus	Hindu women will prefer female doctors.
	Prayer rituals may be continued.
	Dying patients may wish to lie on the floor to be close to 'Earth'.
	Rites including tying of a holy thread and sprinkling with water from the River Ganges. Religious tokens should not be removed.
	Body should not be touched by non-Hindus (if necessary wear gloves) and should be prepared according to the wishes of the family or priest.
	Ideally cremation should be arranged within 24 hours, often not practicable.
	No specific religious objection to postmortem or organ donation although these are not liked.
Sikhs	Sikh women will prefer female doctors.
	Sikh men will wish to keep their hair covered at all times.
	The five symbols of faith should not be disturbed in life or death.
	Running water preferred for washing.
	No specific ceremonial rites at death.
	Traditionally Sikh families will lay out the body but no specific objection to others touching the body.

BASIC PRINCIPLES

INFECTION CONTROL

Patients receiving intensive care are at greatly increased risk of hospital acquired (nosocomial) infections. This is a result of their underlying disease process, which often results in some degree of immune suppression. Drugs such as steroids, multiple lines and tubes which bypass defensive barriers such as mucosal surfaces, add to the problem. Patients are at risk from their own flora, in particular that associated with the gastrointestinal tract, but also from organisms transferred from other patients.

Before entering the unit

Before entering the ICU leave your jacket or white coat outside. White coats in particular tend to be dirty and can carry microbiological flora from one patient to the next. Neck ties also have a habit of dangling in all sorts of places; tuck them out of the way.

If you are going to stay on the ICU all day it is a good idea to wear surgical blues to prevent problems with contamination of clothes. This not only reduces the risk of cross-infection but saves on your laundry bills as well!

Before approaching the patient

Simple measures are the best way to reduce infection risks. Therefore, before you go near a patient in the ICU, you should:

● Put on a disposable plastic apron.
● Wash your hands thoroughly. If your hands are already socially clean you can use an alcohol disinfectant rub which is equally effective.

Do not share equipment between patients in the ICU. For example stethoscopes are generally provided at each bed space. You should not use your own which might be a vehicle for cross- infection.

● Wash your hands again or use alcohol disinfectant rub after each patient that you see, and change your plastic apron.

(Reverse) barrier nursing

Some patients may be at particular risk from infection, because they are immunocompromised as a result of drug therapy, radiotherapy or immune disease including HIV infection. These patients will often be in a side room and barrier nursed to help protect them.

The basic principles of barrier nursing are:

● Do not enter unnecessarily.
● Wear an apron.
● Wash your hands and put on gloves.

Other precautions such as masks and gowns will depend on the particular nature of the problem. Instructions for entering the room are generally displayed on the door, and the nurses will help.

Barrier nursing

Some patients may be isolated because they have a serious infection or are colonized with an antibiotic resistant organism which may be transmitted to other patients or even on occasions to members of staff. The precautions are generally similar to the above:

● Remove protective aprons, etc. before you leave the room.
● Wash your hands after visiting the patient, and before you leave the room.

 Warning! These precautions are in addition to the universal precautions that you should employ when dealing with patient's body fluids. (See Universal precautions p. 226.)

Other aspects of preventing and dealing with infection in the ICU will be dealt with later (See Pneumonia, p. 88 and sepsis p. 199.)

ASSESSING A PATIENT

Each patient in the ICU needs to be seen and assessed at least twice a day. Many conventional aspects of history taking and examination are either inappropriate or impracticable. This can seem daunting to the new trainee, particularly given the large amount of information available from charts, monitors and equipment at the patient's bedside. It is best to work out a system for condensing information easily so that you can assess the patient and work out a plan.

History

Make sure you know the detailed history of the patient. It is particularly important when admitting a new patient to avoid overlooking important facts. Although history may often not be available from the patient, there is generally a lot of information available from the notes, from other doctors, nurses, or the referring hospital. If in doubt, telephone the referring team. Take time to speak to family and friends to ascertain preexisting health, physiological reserve, and attitudes to life support.

Patient's chart

Looking at the patient's chart next is an extension of the history. It can be scanned for general trends in the patient's condition since arrival in intensive care or examined more closely to give a guide to progress over the preceding 24 hours. Important things to note from the chart are:

● Evidence of infection:
  – temperature and white cell count.

- Haemodynamic stability:
  - trends in haemodynamic variables such as pulse, blood pressure, CVP, pulmonary artery pressures, cardiac output, inotrope requirements and evidence of adequate organ perfusion (e.g. conscious level, renal output, lactate).
- Respiratory function:
  - type and mode of ventilation, levels of respiratory support
  - progress made weaning
  - blood gases.
- Gastric and renal function:
  - adequate volume and quality of urine
  - plasma and urinary electrolytes
  - fluid intake
  - nutrition—parenteral or enteral?
  - overall fluid balance.
- CNS function:
  - conscious level, sedation and analgesic requirements.

Examining the patient

Once you have put together the information available from the history and the patient's chart you should examine the patient carefully.

 Warning! Before examining a patient introduce yourself and explain what you are going to do, even if they appear unconscious. Remember that hearing may be the last sense to be lost under anaesthesia or sedation.

You should examine the patient in the normal way. However you will need to assimilate information available from the monitoring at the same time. For example:

- Cardiovascular:
  - pulse, blood pressure, CVP, wedge pressure and cardiac output
  - heart sounds
  - evidence of adequate perfusion
  - cold and sweaty versus warm peripheries
  - temperature gradient
  - peripheral oedema
  - line sites clean or evidence of infection.
- Respiratory:
  - trachea central, air entry bilateral equal, breath sounds, added sounds
  - check position and adequacy of chest drains, endotracheal tubes, etc.
  - check type and adequacy of ventilation and ventilator settings
  - CXR may be considered an extension of the physical examination in intensive care patients.

- Abdomen:
  - soft or tender, distended
  - bowel sounds present
  - bowels open
  - diarrhoea
  - enteral or parenteral feeding.
- Renal:
  - urine output
  - fluid balance.
- CNS:
  - level of consciousness
  - consider stopping all sedative/analgesic drugs to assess neurological status
  - does the patient make purposeful movements of all 4 limbs to command or stimulus?
  - for painful stimulus press on nail bed or supraorbital ridge (other sites cause bruising)
  - intracranial pressure and cerebral perfusion pressure.
- Limbs:
  - adequate perfusion (especially after injury)
  - evidence of swelling, tenderness, DVT, or compartment syndrome.
- Wounds:
  - surgical wounds, and trauma sites, inspection for adequate healing
  - evidence of infection or discharge
  - surgical drains, volume and nature of drainage.

Special investigations
When you have examined the patient, you should go back to the patient's chart and records and check on anything that you have missed. Also review the patient's important haematology, biochemical and microbiology investigations and other investigations including CXRs.

Prescription charts
Review the patient's drug, fluid and nutrition prescription chart. Particularly check that routine stress ulcer prophylaxis and DVT prophylaxis is appropriately prescribed. Are current prescriptions appropriate to the patient's needs? In particular are antibiotics still needed? Do any prescriptions require plasma drug level monitoring? Are any of the prescribed drugs likely to interact?

Daily problem list
When you have recorded your examination findings and any important results in the medical notes, it is useful to summarize your findings by making a brief list of the current problems: For example:

1. Continuing sepsis WCC 34, cause?: central lines 6 days old.
2. Haemodynamically unstable. Increasing inotrope requirements. Adequately filled?
3. Urine output deteriorating, creatinine rising 435: renal referral?

Formulating action plan

Using this approach you can prioritize problems and choose a plan of action. In practice this should be done in consultation with the consultant looking after the ICU. The action plan should include the following.

- Action targeted against problems identified.
- Integrated plan for each organ system requiring support.
- Ventilation and/or weaning plan.
- 24-hour fluid intake and fluid balance including nutrition.
- Drug therapy.
- Further investigations required.

When you have finished with the patient and detailed your findings and plans in the medical notes you should tell the nurses what is planned. In particular:

- Leave detailed instructions and parameters for the manipulation of drugs such as inotropes which are generally titrated to response (i.e. what mean wedge and blood pressure are acceptable).
- Discuss any major changes in therapy or new problems with the referring consultant team.
- Finally, you should keep the relatives informed of progress. (See Talking to relatives, p. 7.)

When using this general approach to help you to formulate a management plan you should consider the following basic principles which are relevant to all patients in the ICU. Notes on particular medical problems can be found in later sections.

SEDATION AND ANALGESIA

The purpose of sedation and analgesia is to make patients comfortable during their stay in the intensive care, while allowing nursing and medical procedures to be performed safely. Comfort encompasses a number of areas of different importance to each patient.

- Tolerance of endotracheal intubation, assisted ventilation, invasive catheters, etc.
- Analgesia (painful wounds, limbs, viscera).
- Unawareness of frightening environment.
- Amnesia for unpleasant procedures.
- Allowing 'natural' sleep patterns.

Problems of over-sedation

There is increasing pressure in ICU facilities and ideally patients should be awake enough for discharge as soon as their physical condition allows. Excessive sedation is undesirable and may result in the following:

- Prolonged need for IPPV/intubation.
- Haemodynamic instability.
- Gastrointestinal tract stasis.
- Potential immune suppression.
- Potential organ toxicity.
- Difficulty in assessing neurological state.

Ideally, once stabilized, patients should be able sit or stand at the bedside despite still being dependant on drugs, dialysis and assisted ventilation. In reality this is difficult to achieve. Optimum care therefore, should aim at an awake, pain-free patient who can move about as much as possible and cooperate with physiotherapy and nursing care.

Sedation scoring systems are a useful guide. Levels 2 to 5 are ideals which are appropriate for most intensive care patients (see Table 2.1).

TABLE 2.1 Sedation score
1. Anxious, agitated, restless
2. Cooperative, orientated, tranquil
3. Responds to commands only
4. Asleep but awakens on light stimulation
5. Asleep sluggish response to stimulation
6. No response
7. Paralysed*
*See Muscle Relaxants below

In practice the requirements for drugs differ markedly between patients. Younger fitter patients require more sedation and analgesia. Patients who abuse alcohol and other centrally acting drugs may be very difficult to sedate owing to cross-tolerance between the abused substance and sedative agents prescribed. Relatives and patients often deny such usage. Acute tolerance to drugs used for sedation in ICU may also occur.

When drugs used before admission, or sedative drugs given in ICU are stopped, drug withdrawal states may develop. This may result in seizures, hallucinations, delirium tremens, confusional states, agitation and aggression. These phenomena are difficult to control without further heavy sedation, but usually settle over time.

Causes of acute confusional state
- Side-effects of prescribed drugs
- Withdrawal of alcohol or other drugs
- Toxic encephalopathy
- Renal and hepatic encephalopathy
- Sleep deprivation (especially REM sleep)
- Elderly patients particularly susceptible

There is little hard data on drug effects on metabolism and excretion in the critically ill. Drug trials performed in rats, healthy 'volunteers', ASA I patients, compensated cirrhosis and uraemia bear little resemblance to the typical ICU patient. Therefore repeated assessment of sedation and analgesia is required. Drugs should be given by bolus or intermittent infusion and consideration should be given to stopping them daily to avoid accumulation and over-sedation.

No single agent is effective alone and combinations of drugs are used (similar to the concept of balanced anaesthesia). The most widely used is a mixture of opioids and benzodiazepines. Fentanyl and alfentanil, although potent analgesics, have less sedative effects than morphine derivatives. Epidural techniques, other regional anaesthetic techniques and patient controlled analgesia (PCA) are very useful in patients with painful wounds.

 Warning! The following notes and drug doses are for guidance only. Choice of drug will depend upon local practice (if in doubt, ask!). Exact doses should be titrated to the individual patient's needs. Use the smallest doses of analgesic and sedative drugs required to achieve the desired effect. For further information refer to BNF or seek senior advice.

Diazepam
(5–10 mg IV bolus)
This is a cheap cardiostable, sedative, amnesic, anticonvulsant which should be considered as a first line sedative, usually by intermittent boluses. It has a long elimination half-life, active metabolites and accumulates in the sicker patient hence is better not given by continuous infusion.

Midazolam
(2–5 mg IV bolus)
(2–10 mg/h by infusion)
A useful alternative to diazepam with similar properties. Although it has a considerably shorter half-life in the healthy patient this is not always the case in the sicker ICU case where its advantages are less clear cut. May be given by continuous infusion but this is associated with a higher incidence of accumulation.

Propofol

(1–3 mg/kg IV bolus for intubation)
(10–20 mg bolus for sedation repeated to effect)
(2–5 mg/kg/h by infusion)
Propofol is an effective anaesthetic, sedative, anticonvulsant, amnesic agent. Its main advantage over other agents is its rapid termination of effects on switching off the infusion. Cost, lipid accumulation and cardiovascular instability are the main disadvantages. Not licensed for infusion in children.

Morphine

(2–5 mg IV bolus)
Standard opiate for intermittent use and PCA systems. Continuous infusions are best avoided to prevent accumulation. Avoid in patients with significant renal impairment (risk of accumulation of active metabolites).

Typical PCAS regimen
50 mg morphine in 50 ml 0.9% saline
1 mg bolus
5-minute lockout time
No background infusion

Fentanyl

(2–6 µg/kg/h by infusion)
(Adults generally 0.1–0.5 mg/h)
Shorter acting than morphine, no active metabolites. No accumulation in renal failure.

Alfentanil

(20–250 µg/kg/h by infusion)
(Adults generally 1–4 mg/h)
Shorter acting than fentanyl, no active metabolites, no accumulation in renal failure. Rapid termination of effects after discontinuation. May be expensive if infused in large doses.

Chlorpromazine (as *Haloperidol* below)

(5–10 mg IV bolus repeated as necessary)

Haloperidol

(5–10 mg IV bolus repeated as necessary)
Chlorpromazine and haloperidol are major tranquillizers; useful agents which calm the patient without undue sedation or respiratory depression. Use in acute confusional states or when other agents are not achieving satisfactory effects in sensible doses. They are potent alpha blockers: beware of hypotension. Give as a slow IV bolus.

Naloxone (as *Flumazenil* on p. 28)

(0.4–2 mg IV bolus repeated as necessary)

Flumazenil

(0.2 mg IV bolus repeated as necessary)

Competitive antagonist of opioid and benzodiazepine receptors respectively, naloxone and flumazenil are useful in occasional cases to reverse respiratory depression, sedation and hypotension caused by opioids and benzodiazepines. Both have short half-life (20 min) leading to recurrence of respiratory depression and sedation. Risk of fits, hypertension, arrhythmias (especially in patients who have taken mixed overdoses). Do not infuse over long periods, ventilate patient and await redistribution and metabolism of drugs!

COMMON PROBLEM: PATIENT DIFFICULT TO SEDATE

If patients are difficult to sedate check that sedative infusions are running correctly and at the prescribed dose. In addition:

● Review other drug therapy and stop where appropriate. Many drugs (for example H_2 blockers) have the potential to induce confusional states.
● Exclude possible causes of agitation including: full bladder, painful wound, hypoxia, hypercarbia, endotracheal tube touching carina.
● Consider the value of tracheostomy over conventional intubation. May be better tolerated and allows sedative and analgesic drugs to be significantly reduced.

Consider alternative cocktail of drugs. Eventually all patients will require to be weaned off drugs and there is often a difficult phase when the patient is partially sedated but unable to cooperate due to residual drug effects. Real problem patients, for example, those post head injury or suffering from withdrawal of drugs or alcohol may be best nursed on a mattress on the floor. This reduces risk of harm should the patient fall out of bed.

COMMON PROBLEM: PATIENT WHO WILL NOT WAKE UP

If a patient fails to regain full consciousness after sedative and analgesic drugs have been stopped for a period of time, the question 'why?' invariably arises. This is usually due to the accumulation of drugs or their active metabolites and resolves with time. A trial of naloxone or flumazenil may be diagnostic. Other causes of coma should also be considered. EEG and CT scan may be helpful. In particular consider:

● Effects of sepsis (for example as part of multiple-organ failure).
● Metabolic derangement.
● Structural brain damage (including CVA, hypoxic brain injury).
● Awake patients who cannot respond ('locked-in syndrome').

MUSCLE RELAXANTS

The routine use of muscle relaxants in ICU is of little proven benefit and their use is declining. Problems include:

● Awareness, when patients are inadequately sedated and are conscious during unpleasant procedures. Beware as increasing numbers of surgical procedures, such as tracheostomy, are performed in ICU!

● Accidental unnoticed disconnections of the ventilator may result in hypoxia because the patient cannot make any respiratory effort.

● Neuropathies and myopathies are common in patients with multiple organ failure and may be exaggerated by the prolonged use of muscle relaxants.

Therefore use should be restricted to the following:

● To facilitate endotracheal intubation.

● The management of patients with brain injury or cerebral oedema (to prevent rises in ICP on coughing).

● The management of patients with extreme cardiovascular or respiratory insufficiency where the balance between oxygen delivery and oxygen consumption may be improved by preventing muscle activity.

The choice of drugs depends upon the requirement and the patient's general condition.

 Warning! The following notes and drug doses are for guidance only. Exact doses will depend upon the requirement and the patient's condition. For further information refer to BNF or seek senior advice.

Suxamethonium
(Intubation: 1 mg/kg IV bolus)
This is a short acting depolarizing muscle relaxant which gives good intubating conditions in less than a minute. It is ideal for rapidly intubating patients in an emergency and has the advantage for the inexperienced anaesthetist that it generally wears off in a couple of minutes so that if intubation is difficult spontaneous respiratory effort can be rapidly re-established. In a small number of patients however, the effects are prolonged because of a genetic abnormality in the cholinesterase enzyme which breaks down suxamethonium.

Suxamethonium may also cause bradycardia. All patients suffer a small rise (0.5–1 mmol/l) in serum potassium following suxamethonium. In some groups of patients however, the rise in potassium is much greater and may result in a cardiac arrest. For these and other reasons some people believe that suxamethonium should not be used on the ICU at all.

Contraindications to suxamethonium
Recent burns or crush injuries
Neurological deficit (e.g. spinal injury)
Renal failure with a raised K^+
Myasthenia gravis
Myotonia

Atracurium
(Intubation 0.5 mg/kg IV bolus)
(Infusion 0.5–1 mg/kg/h)
This is a short acting non-depolarizing muscle relaxant. It can be used for intubation and provided adequate conditions in 1.5–2 minutes. Atracurium undergoes spontaneous degradation and therefore does not accumulate in hepatorenal failure. For this reason it is ideal for use by infusion.

Vecuronium
(Intubation 0.1 mg/kg IV bolus)
(Infusion 0.05–0.2 mg/kg/h)
This is an alternative to the above. It may be associated with bradycardia when used by infusion. Avoid in older more unstable patients with renal or hepatic dysfunction who accumulate parent drug and active metabolites.

Pancuronium
(Intubation 0.1 mg/kg IV bolus)
This may produce tachycardia and an elevation in blood pressure. It is relatively long-acting and accumulates in renal failure. Therefore it is used for intermittent bolus injection and not as an infusion. It may be useful for transferring patients, avoiding the need for infusion.

Monitoring neuromuscular blockade
The use of muscle relaxants should be regularly reviewed and consideration given to stopping them intermittently to assess the adequacy of sedation. Neuromuscular blockade can be monitored if required using nerve stimulators. Typical patterns of response are shown in Figure 2.1.

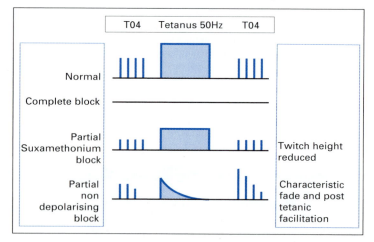

Fig. 2.1 Monitoring neuromuscular function.

Other than for intubation purposes, it is usually unnecessary to completely abolish all muscle response (see Table 2.2) When using non-depolarizing muscle relaxants by infusion, 75–90% block is usually adequate. This equates to 1 or 2 twitches present on a train of four.

TABLE 2.2 Summary of sedation and analgesic regimens

Analgesia	Morphine by bolus Alfentanil/fentanyl by bolus or infusion
Sedation	Diazepam by bolus or Midazolam by bolus or infusion or Propofol by infusion
Relaxants (when indicated)	Atracurium/vecuronium by bolus and/or infusion

PSYCHOLOGICAL CARE

It is stressful to be a patient in intensive care. Despite sedation and analgesia patients are not anaesthetized and may be aware of their surroundings during their stay. Even the sickest patient who may be heavily sedated at the height of their illness will hopefully go on to a period of convalescence, when they will be fully aware of their surroundings. A number of factors may contribute to patient's distress.

Environment
The ICU is a very noisy place and often the only lighting is artificial. Patients may spend long periods in the same room with little knowledge of the outside world. Even the appreciation of day and night may be lost resulting in disturbed sleep patterns. In addition sedative drugs abolish rapid eye movement (dream) sleep and this can cause marked psychological disturbance particularly during the convalescent stage.

Communication difficulties
Communication difficulties following tracheal intubation have not been adequately resolved. Written messages and letter boards are cumbersome, and lip reading is often difficult. Speaking aids for ventilated patients are available in the form of an artificial larynx to produce tones, but none is satisfactory for acute use as they take time and practice to work well.

Dependency
Patients in intensive care are totally dependent both on the nursing staff for their personal needs and on machines and drugs. In addition they may be repeatedly visited by large groups of doctors, and other staff. This is humiliating and depersonalizing.

Pain, fear and anxiety

Many patients in intensive care will have painful surgical wounds and almost all will be subjected to repeated, potentially painful, procedures. Patients may be aware how sick they are or that are possibly dying. The overall experience is very frightening.

To reduce the impact of these problems think about psychological care of your patient.

In particular:

● Take time to get to know patients. Acknowledge their fears and anxieties. Give appropriate explanations and reassurance.
● Respect patient privacy as much as possible.
● Avoid unnecessarily large ward rounds and talking over the patient.
● Always explain procedures to patients and provide adequate analgesia or anaesthesia.
● Avoid disturbing the patient at night if possible. Encourage day-time stimulation in the form of visits from relatives and children, television and radio all of which improve morale.

Despite every effort some patients develop apparent psychoses which require treatment. Others (particularly long-stay patients) may become markedly depressed and withdrawn. Consideration should be given to appropriate antidepressant therapy although there are arguments against their use in so-called reactive depression. Amitriptyline at night may aid nocturnal sleep and help to elevate mood and motivation.

FLUIDS AND ELECTROLYTES

The management of fluids and electrolyte balance in critically ill patients is fundamental to intensive care. Under normal circumstances daily input and output are in balance and the figures (in ml) are approximately as shown in Figure 2.2.

This corresponds to daily requirements of:

water:	30–35 ml/kg/d
Na^+	1–1.5 mmol/kg/d
K^+	1 mmol/kg/d

Thus requirements could be provided by 2 to 3 litres of 4% dextrose and 0.18% saline with additional potassium 20 mmol per litre. However for the critically ill patient on the intensive care unit the situation is more complex owing to the conditions below.

Reduced fluid requirement

● Stress response to critical illness. Increased activity of the renin–angiotensin–aldosterone axis results in reduced sodium excretion. At the same time increased secretion of antidiuretic hormone (ADH) reduces secretion of free water.
● Oliguric renal failure.

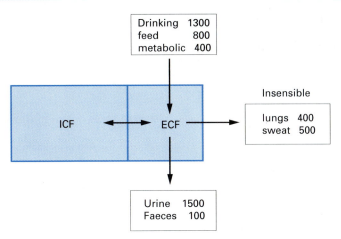

Fig. 2.2 Fluid balance.

Increased fluid requirement

● Gastrointestinal tract dysfunction.
● Wide spread capillary leak associated with sepsis and inflammatory conditions may result in redistribution of body water out of the vascular compartment, and the development of pulmonary and peripheral oedema.
● Burns, skin loss.
● Insensible losses may be increased by poor humidification of inspired ventilator gases. Pyrexia may be associated with substantial losses as sweat. Losses may occur as a result of diarrhoea and there may be additional losses from wounds and drains, etc.
● Underlying condition, effects of multiple procedures and venesections. This may require repeated blood transfusions. Significant coagulopathy may require use of other blood products such as fresh frozen plasma (FFP) and platelet concentrates.

Practical fluid management

● Measure 24-hour fluid balance accurately. The nurses will chart the totals of all fluids in and out of the patients on an hourly basis. This will include all intravenous and nasogastric fluids, all drugs and all measurable losses. It does not include unmeasurable insensible losses, nor shifts in and out of the vascular space.
● Measure plasma electrolytes frequently. Sodium (Na^+) and potassium (K^+) at least every 4–6 hours. Magnesium (Mg^{2+}) Calcium (Ca^{2+}) and Phosphate (PO_4^{3-}) daily or as required.
● Additional measurements such as plasma and urinary osmolality and urinary electrolytes are useful in difficult cases. (See 'Oliguria', p. 120.)

The aim is to keep the patient hydrated, with an adequate circulating volume and normal electrolytes. Exact fluid regimens will depend on the patient's clinical state of hydration, (look at tongue, mucous membranes, tissue turgor, urine output) cumulative fluid balance on the charts, and electrolyte investigations.

A typical fluid regimen for a 70-kg adult patient (not receiving nutritional support) will be:

● Crystalloid: Dextrose 4% and saline 0.18% @ 80–120 ml/h. Plus 20–60 mmol K^+ per litre.
● Additional K^+ (20 mmol in 20 ml 0.9% saline) as required to maintain normal potassium.
● Additional Ca^{2+}, Mg^{2+} and phosphate as required.
● Colloids as additionally required to maintain adequate central venous filling pressures.
● Blood products as additionally required.

With this sort of regimen it is possible to render patients fluid-overloaded as measured by positive fluid balance and generalized oedema, despite apparently only maintaining adequate filling pressures. This generally resolves as the patient's condition improves. However, you should review the fluid balance and regimen regularly and adjust it as seems necessary. If in doubt consider a fluid challenge or trial of diuretics. Low-dose diuretics (for example 10–20 mg frusemide will often produce a good diuresis in the overloaded patient but have little effect or toxicity in others). (See Oliguria, p. 120.)

Disturbances of fluid and electrolyte balance are discussed further in the section on metabolism.

NUTRITION

During the acute phase of illness, intensive care patients are generally catabolic. Muscle is broken down to provide amino acids for energy requirements and for synthesis of acute phase proteins. Nitrogen from protein breakdown is lost in the urine and patients develop a negative nitrogen balance. This may result in severe muscle wasting and weakness, greatly prolonging recovery. The aim of feeding patients is therefore to provide adequate amino acids and energy to minimize this process.

Assessment of nutritional status

When examining patients in the ICU it is worth noting their nutritional status in terms of muscle bulk. Note that wasting may often be hidden by oedema fluid and it is only on recovery, when oedema fluids shift, that the true extent of wasting is visible. It is reasonable to assume all critically ill patients are at risk of established or impending nutritional deficiency, hence the urgent need for nutritional replacement.

Nutrition can be provided by the enteral or parenteral route depending upon the circumstances (see below). Whichever route is chosen the aim is to provide all the patient's nutritional requirements. In particular those listed below.

Water
30–35 ml/kg/d
In addition losses, for example, increased insensible losses associated with rise in temperature. Add 150 ml per day per 1°C rise in temperature.

Electrolytes

Na⁺	1–1.5 mmol/kg/d	(100 mmol)
K⁺	1 mmol/kg/d	(60–80 mmol)
Phosphate	0.5 mmol/kg/d	(<50 mmol)

Energy
Energy requirements depend on body mass, and metabolic rate.

Normally 30–40–Kcal/kg/d

Increased in critical illness >55 Kcal/kg/d

This can be estimated from various formulae: For example; see Table 2.3

TABLE 2.3 Schofield equation		
Age (years)	**Male**	**Female**
15–18	BMR = $17.6 \times$ weight (kg) + 656	BMR = $13.3 \times$ weight (kg) + 690
18–30	BMR = $15.0 \times$ weight (kg) + 690	BMR = $14.8 \times$ weight (kg) + 485
30–60	BMR = $11.4 \times$ weight (kg) + 870	BMR = $8.1 \times$ weight (kg) + 842
> 60	BMR = $11.7 \times$ weight (kg) + 585	BMR = $9.0 \times$ weight (kg)+ 656

Determination of energy requirements
To BMR add:

1. Stress factor:
+10–30% severe sepsis, +10–30% extensive surgery, +10–30% fractures and trauma, +50–150% burns, +20% ARDS
2. Energy requirements above BMR
+20% immobile, +30% bed bound but not immobile, +40% mobile on ward
3. +10% for metabolic effect of food
4. Temperature factor. +10% for each 1°C rise in temperature

An alternative method of estimating energy requirements is indirect calorimetry. A number of 'metabolic computers' are now available which sample the patient's inspired and expired gases and using an assumed value for the respiratory quotient can estimate total energy expenditure. Energy requirements are generally provided as a mixture of carbohydrate and fats.

Nitrogen (protein)

To prevent muscle breakdown adequate amounts of nitrogen must be provided. This is generally of the order of 9–14 g of nitrogen a day, equivalent to 1–2 g protein/kg/day. Proteins should be provided in a form that ensures that all the essential amino acids are provided. There is increasing interest in the role of individual amino acids. For example, glutamine has a specific role as a substrate for metabolism within the gastrointestinal tract where it is important in maintaining integrity and function.

Minerals and trace elements

Tables of requirements for trace elements and minerals are available, including calcium, magnesium, iron, zinc, copper, selenium, molybdenum, manganese and chromium. Many of these have important roles in enzyme pathways and as free radical scavengers.

Vitamins

Both water and fat soluble vitamins can be provided by commercially available preparations. Folic acid and vitamin B_{12} should be prescribed separately.

ENTERAL FEEDING

Enteral feeding is the preferred means of nutritional support. Advice should be sought from the dietician for exact nutritional requirements, however, ready to use off-the-shelf enteral feeding formulae are available and are suitable for most patients.

Therefore do not wait for specialist dietician advice before starting enteral feed. Start empirical feeds out of hours and seek a tailored approach on the next working day. It is unnecessary in intubated patients to stop feeds for repeated surgical procedures like daily pack changes or tracheostomy.

Indications

Unless there is a specific surgical contraindication, all patients should receive enteral feeding as soon as possible, preferably within 24 hours. This provides nutrition and helps to maintain gastrointestinal tract integrity and function. (See Stress ulcer prophylaxis, p. 39 and Gastrointestinal tract, p. 108.)

Contraindications

Contraindications include paralytic ileus, intestinal obstruction, and surgical conditions of the oesophagus or abdomen.

 Warning! The absence of bowel sounds alone in a ventilated patient without other evidence of ileus should not prevent attempts to commence enteral feeding.

Route of administration

The majority of patients in the ICU will already have a large bore nasogastric tube in situ for gastric aspiration. This can be used for short-term feeding. In patients who require longer term feeding and who are convalescing, fine bore nasogastric feeding tubes are more comfortable and less likely to cause mucosal erosions. (See Practical procedures, p. 263.)

Delayed gastric emptying is a major factor limiting the success of enteral feeding. There is increasing interest in the use of feeding tubes placed through the pylorus which deliver enteral feed directly into the duodenum or jejunum. These can be placed using X-ray screening or endoscopic techniques. The use of percutaneous endoscopic gastrostomy (PEG) is increasing. These have the advantage of removing all nasogastric tubes which can increase the risks of nosocomial infection.

Feeding regimen

Continuous infusion of enteral feed over 24 hours is the usual method. Once feeding is well established it is common to rest the patient for 4 hours in every 24 (often overnight) to allow the gastric pH to return to normal (acid) levels. This helps to prevent colonization of the stomach with gastrointestinal tract flora which is associated with an increased incidence of nosocomial pneumonia.

Many units have policies for commencing enteral feeding. For example:

- Commence enteral feed at 30 ml/hour.
- Give feed for 4 hours followed by 1 hour's rest.
- Aspirate NG tube to assess gastric residual volume.
- If feed absorbed increase in 25 ml increments every 5 hours up to 100 ml/hour.

Complications of enteral feeding

Complications of enteral feeding

- Tube malposition or displacement.
- Tube occlusion.
- Abdominal cramps and bloating.
- Regurgitation pulmonary aspiration.
- Diarrhoea.
- Increased risk of nosocomial infection associated with NG tubes.
- Metabolic derangement.

COMMON PROBLEM: FEED NOT ABSORBED

High gastric residual volume suggests enteral feed is not being absorbed (gastroparesis, etc.). If after 4 hour's feed and 1 hour's rest the gastric residual volume is more than 50% of administered feed, do not increase feeding rate. Continue for another 4 hours at the same rate and then reassess. If the feed is not absorbed consider the use of prokinetic drugs to promote gastric emptying.

- Metoclopramide 10 mg IV 8 hourly.
- Cisapride 10 mg orally or rectally 8 hourly.

If feed is still not absorbed, consider further investigation such as plain abdominal X-ray to exclude obstruction. Unless there is a contraindication to feeding do not stop attempts at enteral feeding. Continue at a low rate, for example 10–20 ml/hour.

COMMON PROBLEM: MANAGEMENT OF DIARRHOEA

Diarrhoea commonly complicates enteral feeding in the ICU. The causes of this are multifactorial. Diarrhoea is generally a nuisance rather than a serious problem, however it may result in the need to abandon enteral feeding.

- Do not immediately stop enteral feed. Discuss with the dietician changing the feed to reduce the osmolarity and increase the fibre content.
- Confirm diarrhoea is not infective in nature: send stool specimens for microscopy and culture (*Salmonella*, *Shigella* and *Campylobacter* species) and for *Clostridium difficile* toxin.
- Treat any infective process appropriately. For *Clostridium difficile* use oral or nasogastric metronidazole or vancomycin.
- Review the drug chart. Stop any prokinetic drugs such as metoclopramide or cisapride. If the diarrhoea is non-infective consider the use of loperamide.
- If the diarrhoea is bloody or if the nature is unclear consider the need for surgical investigation, e.g. sigmoidoscopy or colonoscopy.
- Perform a rectal examination to exclude faecal impaction (common in elderly) which may be a cause of overflow diarrhoea. Consider suppositories or manual evacuation.

TOTAL PARENTERAL NUTRITION (TPN)

If enteral feeding is contraindicated or cannot be established then TPN may be indicated. It is generally started if the patient is not likely to be able to recommence enteral feeding within a few days, unless the patient is already severely catabolic. If in doubt seek senior advice.

Practical TPN

Most units now use one or two standard mixture feeds, prepared under sterile conditions in the pharmacy or bought in from an outside supplier (Table 2.4.)

TABLE 2.4 Typical standard TPN mixture	
Volume	2.5 litres
Nitrogen source (9–14 g nitrogen)	L–amino acid solution
Energy source (1500–2000 Kcal)	Glucose and lipid emulsion
Additives	Electrolytes, trace elements, vitamins
Other additives	Insulin and H_2 blockers may be added

Few acute patients need regimens specifically tailored to their needs. Patients in renal failure who are not on renal support require a reduced volume and nitrogen intake is restricted to avoid rises in plasma urea. For most patients, however, a standard feed can be started and advice subsequently sought from dieticians, pharmacists or a parenteral feeding team.

In practice decide what volume of feed the patient will tolerate. Standard adult feeds are usually 2.5 litres a day, but can be reduced for fluid restricted patients.

Parenteral feeds are hypertonic and cause thrombophlebitis. They should only be given via central venous lines. When inserting multiple lumen central lines, keep one lumen clean for TPN. Parenteral nutrition mixtures make good culture mediums for bacteria, so do not break the line to give any thing else. TPN is given by constant infusion over 24 hours and delivered by volumetric infusion pumps.

Monitoring of TPN

Advice should be sought from the nutrition team and dieticians. The following should be assessed daily:

● Fluid balance.
● Urea, electrolytes, phosphate, glucose. Blood sugar will often rise and require the addition of an insulin infusion.
● Adequate energy requirements. Judged by degree of catabolism clinically. Nitrogen balance can be calculated but in practice rarely is.
● Liver function (albumin, transferrin and enzymes) indicate adequate protein synthesis and give an early indication of TPN related complications.

Complications

The complications of TPN include all complications of central venous access (See Practical procedures, p. 231). Metabolic derangement particularly hyper- or hypoglycaemia, hypophosphataemia, and hypercalcaemia are not uncommon and require appropriate adjustment of the feed. Hepatobiliary dysfunction, including elevation of hepatic enzymes, jaundice and fatty infiltration of the liver may occur. This is caused by a combination of the patients underlying disease processes and lipid load. It may become necessary to stop TPN or reduce the fat content.

STRESS ULCER PROPHYLAXIS

Early enteral feeding helps to maintain gastrointestinal mucosal blood flow, and provides essential nutrients to the mucosa. Early feeding is therefore important in reducing the incidence of both septic complications and stress ulceration. (See Gastrointestinal tract, p. 108.)

If enteral feeding cannot be established patients should receive alternative prophylactic measures to prevent stress ulceration. For example:

- Sucralfate 1 g NG 6 hourly.
- Ranitidine 50 mg IV 8 hourly.

Histamine (H_2 receptor) blocking drugs such as ranitidine, raise intragastric pH. This is associated with an increased colonization of the upper gastrointestinal tract with lower gastrointestinal tract bacteria and a subsequent increase in the incidence of nosocomial infection. Therefore sucralfate, which acts as a protective barrier to the gastric mucosa without altering intragastric pH is the preferred agent for stress ulcer prophylaxis.

DEEP VENOUS THROMBOSIS (DVT) PROPHYLAXIS

Patients requiring intensive care are at risk for the development of DVT and pulmonary embolism (PE). Causes include immobility, venous stasis, poor circulation, major surgery, malignancy and pre-existing illness. Over and above these well-known factors, intensive care itself is an independent risk factor. Upper limb venous thrombosis is more common in ITU than in other settings usually due to thrombosis following subclavian vein catheterization.

Despite all these risk factors there has been surprisingly little research performed to document either the true incidence of DVT or PE in such a population or what constitutes the best form of prophylaxis. The use of compression stockings and early mobilization of the patients may help to reduce the risk. Once coagulation profiles are within normal ranges low-dose subcutaneous heparin should be given. For example:

- Heparin 5000 units s.c. bd.
- Enoxaparin 20 mg s.c. daily.

Low molecular weight heparins (e.g. enoxaparin) may be associated with a lower incidence of haemorrhage than conventional heparin. Suspected DVT can be confirmed by ultrasound or venography. If confirmed the patient should than be fully anticoagulated initially with heparin and then warfarin when conditions allow.

APACHE SCORING

(See Prediction of outcome, p. 5.)
There has been a great deal of interest in trying to predict the risk of mortality of individual patients from measures of severity of illness, pre-existing disease processes, underlying medical diagnoses and age of patient. The best known of these is APACHE II (Table 2.5).

You may be expected to calculate scores on your patients, usually within 24 hours of admission.

TABLE 2.5 APACHE II: Acute Physiological And Chronic Health Evaluation Score Sheet

Score	+4	+3	+2	+1	0	+1	+2	+3	+4
Temperature°C (core)	>41	39–40.9		38.5–38.9	36–38.4	34–35.9	32–33.9	30–31.9	<29
Resp. rate	>50	35–49		25–34	12–24	10–11	6–9		<5
MAP	>160	130–159	110–129		79–109		55–69	40–54	<39
Oxygen If Fio$_2$>0.5 use A-a gradient	>66.6	46.7–66.5	26.7–46.5		<26.7				
If Fio$_2$<0.5 use PaO$_2$ in Kpa					>9.3	8.1–9.3		7.3–8.0	<7.3
Serum HCO$_3$ mmol/l	>52	41–51.9		32–40.9	22–31.9		18–21.9	15–17.9	<15
or arterial pH	>7.7	7.6–7.69		7.5–7.59	7.33–7.49		7.25–7.32	7.15–7.24	<7.15
Sodium mmol/l	>180	160–179	155–159	150–154	130–153		120–129	111–119	<110
Potassium mmol/l	>7	6–6.9		5.5–5.9	3.5–5.4	3–3.4	2.5–2.9		<2.5
Creatinine µmol/l (double if ARF)	>309	169–306	125–168		53–124		<53		
Hb g/dl	>20		16.7–19.9	16.6–15.4	15.3–10		9.9–6.7		<6.7
White blood count (1000s)	>40		20–39.9	15–19.9	3–14.9		1–2.9		<1
Glasgow Coma Scale				Score 15 minus actual GCS					

Age points (Table 2.6)

TABLE 2.6 Age points

Age	44	45–54	55–64	65–74	75
Score	0	2	3	5	6

Chronic health points

If the patient has a history of severe organ system insufficiency or is immunocompromised assign points as follows:

1. For non-operative or emergency postoperative patients score 5 points *or*
2. For elective postoperative patients score 2 points.

Definitions

Organ insufficiency or immunocompromised state must have been evident prior to this hospital admission and conform to the following criteria.

CVS New York Heart Association Class IV.

Respiratory Chronic restrictive, obstructive or vascular disease resulting in severe exercise restriction, i.e. unable to climb stairs or perform household duties, or documented chronic hypoxia, hypercapnia, secondary polycythaemia, severe pulmonary hypertension or respiratory dependency.

Renal Receiving chronic dialysis.

Liver Biopsy proven cirrhosis and documented portal hypertension, episodes of past upper GI bleeding attributed to portal hypertension or prior episodes of hepatic failure/encephalopathy/coma.

Immunocompromised The patient has received therapy that suppresses resistance to infection, e.g. immunosuppression, chemotherapy, radiation, long-term or recent high-dose steroids, or has a disease that is sufficiently advanced to suppress resistance to infection, e.g. leukaemia, lymphoma, AIDS.

Notes on completing APACHE II scores

APACHE II score = sum of acute physiology + age + chronic health scores.

● Score the worst value for each parameter in the first 24 hours.
● Where results are not available score as zero. But this does not mean that you do not have to try to find the result first!

Oxygen

$Fio_2 > 0.5$. To score this requires calculation of the Alveolar–arterial oxygen difference or $(A–a)Do_2$ expressed in kPa

$$\text{Alveolar Oxygen} = Fio_2 \times (\text{atms.p.}–\text{SVP water})–Paco_2$$
$$A = Fio_2 \times (101–6.2)–Paco_2$$

therefore
$$(A–a)Do_2 = (Fio_2 \times 94.8)–Paco_2–Pao_2$$

The result of this gives the A–a gradient which is then scored from the APACHE table

score	+4	+3	+2	+1	0
result	>66.6	46.7–66.5	26.7–46.5		<26.7

$Fio_2 < 0.5$ Simply score the resulting Pao_2 in kPa.

Score	0	+13	+2	+3	+4
Pao_2(kPa)	>9.3	8.1–9.3		7.3–8.0	<7.15

Serum HCO₃

Only use bicarbonate when there are no blood gases available. Otherwise score the arterial pH.

Glasgow Coma Scale (GCS)

A number of approaches to this are adopted in different units. Commonly, *either* (a) assign the assumed GCS patient would have if not artifically sedated, *or* (b) as patients who are ventilated, paralyzed and sedated, will have a GCS of 3, score as $15 - 3 = 12$ (see below). Ask what is the usual practice in your unit.

Chronic health points

This can provide a significant loading to an APACHE score. Apply only according to the criteria on the scoring chart which imply established organ system impairment.

Problems with APACHE II score

There are a number of problems with the APACHE II score:

● Patients with an APACHE II score >35 are unlikely to survive. However, the score is a statistical tool based on the population and scores for individuals cannot be used to predict outcome. Some patients, for example, those with diabetic ketoacidosis, may have marked physiological abnormalities, but generally get better quickly.
● The score is based on historical data, and as new interventions are developed the data becomes obsolete.
● Lead time bias results from the stabilization of patients in referring hospital prior to transfer. This artificially lowers the score for the patient arriving at the referral centre.
● The GCS component is difficult to assess in the heavily sedated or paralyzed patient. There is a big difference between GCS 3 due to head injury and due to the effects of drugs.
● The physiological components are based on adults. They do not translate to paediatrics. For children the 'Prism' score is usually used instead.

APACHE III score

The APACHE II score has now been superseded by an updated APACHE III score. Five new variables have been added (urine output, serum albumin, urea, bilirubin, and glucose), while two variables (potassium and bicarbonate) have been removed. In addition the Glasgow Coma Scale and acid base balance components have been altered. A complex matrix grid scoring system is used with a maximum score of 299.

OTHER SCORING SYSTEMS

SAPS Score

The Simplified Acute Physiology Score is similar scoring to APACHE and is used more commonly in mainland Europe. It utilizes 12 physiological variables assigned a score according to the degree of derangement.

TISS Score

The Therapeutic Intervention Score System assigns a value to each procedure performed in the ICU. The implication is that the more procedures that are performed on a patient, the sicker they are. It is dependant on the doctor, however, since different physicians will have different thresholds for carrying out many procedures. The score is, therefore, not good for comparing outcome between patients or between different units but is useful as a general guide to the type of care and resources likely to be needed by patients on an individual unit.

CARDIOVASCULAR SYSTEM

DEFINITION OF SHOCK

The optimization of haemodynamic status is a fundamental goal of intensive care. The maintenance of an adequate blood pressure is important for the perfusion of vital organs such as the brain and kidneys. However, the primary role of the cardiovascular system is to deliver oxygenated blood to the tissues. When this mechanism fails, shock ensues.

Shock is a syndrome of cardiovascular system failure encompassing tissue hypoperfusion with relative hypotension. This can result in end organ failure, and is a leading cause of prolonged ICU stay.

TABLE 3.1 Causes of shock

Direct cause	Underlying cause
Hypovolaemia	Dehydration
	Haemorrhage
	Burns
	Sepsis
Cardiogenic	Myocardial infarction/ischaemia
	Valve disruption
	Myocardial rupture (VSD, etc.)
Mechanical/obstructive	PE
	Tamponade
	Tension pneumothorax
Altered systemic vascular resistance	Sepsis
	Anaemia
	Anaphylaxis
	Addisionian crisis

The aetiology of shock is multifactorial (see Table 3.1). Apart from mechanical causes, the management of these is similar. You should understand factors which affect oxygen delivery and oxygen consumption.

OXYGEN DELIVERY AND OXYGEN CONSUMPTION

Oxygen delivery (DO$_2$)

Oxygen delivery is defined as the total amount of oxygen delivered to the tissues per minute. It depends on the cardiac output (CO) and the oxygen content of arterial blood as shown.

$$DO_2 = CO \times [\text{arterial oxygen content}]$$
$$DO_2 = CO \times [SaO_2 \times Hb^* \times 1.34) + (\text{dissolved oxygen})]$$

Ignoring dissolved oxygen which is insignificant at atmospheric pressure typical figures are:

$$1000 \text{ ml/min} = 5000 \text{ ml} \times 99/100 \times 15/100 \times 1.34$$

Hb* = haemoglobin g/dl (divide by 100 for g/ml)
1.34 = amount of oxygen (ml) bound to 1 g of fully saturated haemoglobin.

Oxygen consumption (VO₂)

Oxygen consumption is the total amount of oxygen consumed by the tissues per minute. It can be calculated from the difference in oxygen content of arterial and mixed venous blood.

$$VO_2 = CO \times [(\text{arterial oxygen content})-(\text{mixed venous oxygen content})]$$
$$VO_2 = CO \times [(SaO_2 \times Hb \times 1.34)-(S\bar{v}O_2{}^* \times Hb \times 1.34)]$$

*$S\bar{v}O_2$ measured from blood drawn from distal lumen of pulmonary artery catheter.

If cardiac index is used in the above calculations (see below), then oxygen delivery and oxygen consumption can also be expressed as an index. Typical normal values at rest are:

DO_2	1000 ml/min	DO_2L	550 ml/min/m²
VO_2	250 ml/min	VO_2L	150 ml/min/m²

As can be seen the normal oxygen consumption by the tissue is only about 25% of the oxygen delivered. This provides a large margin for safety, so that if oxygen requirements go up, for example in exercise, more oxygen can be extracted and utilized.

In disease states oxygen requirements are often raised, but the ability of the tissues to extract and utilize oxygen may be impaired. Under these circumstances, tissue utilization of oxygen may become limited by the available supply. In order to prevent tissue hypoxia and organ dysfunction, oxygen delivery must be increased.

Optimizing oxygen delivery

● Ensure adequate arterial oxygen saturation.
● Give blood to optimize haemoglobin. Ideally Hb should be raised to 15 g/dl. However, this is associated with an increase in blood viscosity and may result in worsening tissue perfusion and oxygen delivery. In most cases a Hb of 10–12 g/dl is considered optimal. (See Management of the Postoperative patient, p. 212).
● Optimize cardiac output. Fluids and inotropes (See Optimizing haemodynamic status, p. 49).
● If oxygen delivery remains critical, oxygen demand can be reduced by the use of muscle relaxants to reduce the muscle utilization of oxygen.

Continuous mixed venous oxygen saturation ($S\bar{v}O_2$) monitoring using a fibreoptic pulmonary artery catheter gives a useful guide to the balance between oxygen delivery and oxygen consumption. The normal $S\bar{v}O_2$ is 75%. Levels above this imply adequate oxygen delivery and levels below inadequate oxygen delivery. This may be more complicated in those patients with adequate DO_2 who are unable to extract oxygen (sepsis, metabolic poisons, etc.)

Warning! Despite adequate global oxygen delivery as described above, the distribution of blood flow around the body may still result in some tissues receiving an inadequate oxygen delivery. The splanchnic circulation for example is at particular risk of hypoperfusion. (See GIT failure, Sepsis & gastric tonometry pp. 108, 199, 264.)

CARDIAC OUTPUT (CO)

Assuming that oxygen saturation and haemoglobin are adequate, then CO is the main determinant of oxygen delivery. CO is defined as the volume of blood ejected by the heart per minute. In order to take account of the patient's size, it is usually expressed as cardiac index (CI) which is the CO divided by the patient's body surface area (BSA). This is calculated from nomograms. The patient's height and weight are entered and the BSA is calculated by the CO monitoring system.

The factors which affect CO are discussed below. CO is the product of heart rate and stroke volume (SV) (CO = HR × SV).

Heart rate

In a healthy heart and within the physiological range of 70–160 beats per minute, changes in heart rate have little effect on SV. Therefore, an increase in heart rate results in an increase in CO. Critically ill patients tolerate a much narrower range of heart rates, values outside 100–120/min resulting in compromise.

At high rates, SV falls substantially so that CO falls. Tachycardias associated with abnormalities of cardiac rhythm (e.g. atrial fibrillation) further reduce ventricular filling and CO. Tachycardias also increase myocardial oxygen consumption whilst at the same time reducing the time for diastolic perfusion of the ventricles. In patients with ischaemic heart disease, this may produce significant myocardial ischaemia, which may further compromise CO.

Stroke volume (SV)

SV is determined by preload, contractility and afterload.

Preload

This is defined as the ventricular wall tension at the end of diastole. In simple terms preload refers to the degree of ventricular filling. According to the Frank–Starling law of the heart, the greater the degree of ventricular filling, the greater the force of myocardial contraction and thus SV. Above a certain point, however, the ventricle becomes over-stretched and further filling may result in a fall in SV. Heart failure and pulmonary oedema may then develop (see Fig. 3.1).

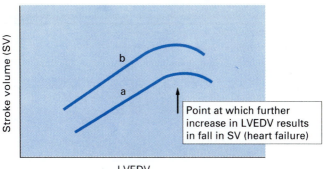

Fig. 3.1 Diagramatic representation of Starling curves: a. Increasing cardiac output as LVEDV increases; b. Effect of increased contractility (inotropes).

Contractility

This represents the ability of the heart to work independent of the preload and afterload. Increased contractility, as, for example produced by inotropes, results in increased SV for the same preload (see Fig. 3.1). Decreased contractility may result from intrinsic heart disease, or from the myocardial depressant effects of acidosis, hypoxia and disease processes, e.g. sepsis.

Afterload

This is defined as the ventricular wall tension at the end of systole. In simple terms this is a measure of the load against which the heart is working. It is increased by ventricular dilatation, outflow resistance (for example, aortic valve stenosis) and increases in the peripheral vascular resistance.

OPTIMIZING HAEMODYNAMIC STATUS

Optimization of haemodynamic status may be of benefit either in the critically ill patient or in the high-risk patient undergoing major surgery. This encompasses both maintenance of CO and oxygen delivery and also maintenance of adequate organ perfusion pressure or blood pressure.

Whilst some information on the likely cardiovascular status of the patient can be obtained from simple clinical examination (peripheral temperature, pulse, blood pressure, urine output, etc.) use of pulmonary artery catheterization, to measure CO and pulmonary artery occlusion pressure (PAOP), may be valuable to guide therapy. (See Practical procedures p. 240: see also Table 3.2.)

TABLE 3.2 Normal values for common measured and calculated parameters

Central venous pressure (CVP)	4–10 mmHg
Pulmonary artery occlusion pressure (PAOP)	5–15 mmHg
Cardiac output (CO)	4–6 l/min
Cardiac index (CI)*	2.5–3.5 l/min/m²
Stroke volume (SV)	60–90 ml/beat
Stroke volume index (SVI)	33–47 ml/beat
Systemic vascular resistance (SVR)	900–1200 dyne.sec./cm⁵
Systemic vascular resistance index (SVRI)	1700–2400 dyne.sec./cm⁵/m²

*CI = CO/BSA.
Other indices (SVRI, PVRI, etc.) calculated using CI

Optimization of the haemodynamic status of the patient will depend upon the exact nature of the clinical picture (See Cardiogenic shock, p. 70 septic shock, p. 201.) The normal values quoted are a guide only and are not necessarily adequate for the patient. There has been great interest in the manipulation of these variables, often to supranormal values, in the belief that it might improve outcomes.

Goal directed therapy

Shoemaker has suggested aiming at cardiac index (4.5 l/min/m²) oxygen delivery index (650 ml/min/m²) and oxygen consumption index (165 ml/min/m²). The evidence that this improves outcome is still debatable. Additionally the indications for and value of pulmonary artery catheterization and related technologies, are hotly debated.

Avoid, therefore, aiming at absolute numbers, use them as a guide only and think in terms of achieving adequate haemodynamic performance for the individual patient. A rational approach is to optimize fluid status and then add an inotrope or vasoconstrictors as required. This is summarized in Fig. 3.2.

OPTIMIZE FILLING STATUS

The optimal filling status for a patient is that which achieves the maximal CO whilst at the same time avoiding any deterioration in gas exchange due to the development of pulmonary oedema. (If this can not be achieved then assisted ventilation may be required.)

● Give fluid according to a predetermined CVP or PAOP, typically 8–10 mmHg if myocardial failure or lung injury, 14–18 mmHg otherwise.

These numbers are somewhat arbitrary and individual patients may require a very different approach – echocardiography is often of value in determining filling status.

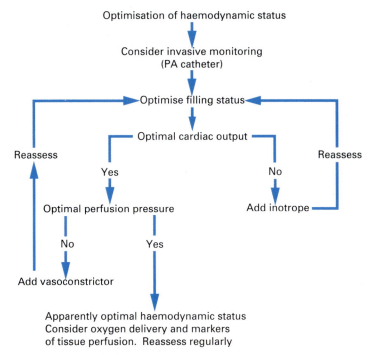

Fig. 3.2 Optimization of haemodynamic status.

Assessment of filling involves measurement of pressure in the right atrium (CVP) or left atrium (PAOP), when what we are really interested in – from Starling Curve – is ventricular end-diastolic volume. The relationship between pressure and volume is complex and involves compliance, which varies with individuals and also with different disease states. It is better, rather than to aim at a specific CVP or PAOP to try and determine the filling pressure which produces the best haemodynamic response from an individual patient. Therefore an alternative approach is:

● Give fluid to increase the CVP or PAOP in small increments and measure the increase in CO or SV. Continue until there is no further improvement or until there is deterioration in arterial blood gases or evidence of pulmonary oedema. (Note: stroke volume index of 50 ml/m² represents a full ventricle.)
● Remember also, that optimal filling may actually mean use of fluid restriction, diuretics and vasodilators to reduce preload in patients with heart failure.

OPTIMIZE CO

Echocardiography

In all but the simplest cases of circulatory failure consider an echocardiogram to establish diagnosis and exclude treatable mechanical causes. Transthoracic and transoesophageal echocardiography give useful information on structural and functional cardiac abnormalities, including pericardial collections, valvular lesions and contractility. Filling, regional wall motion abnormalities and an estimate of flows/pressures can also be made.

Inotropic support

If despite optimal filling CO remains inadequate, inotropes may be added to improve cardiac performance. The rational use of inotropes requires an understanding of the receptor pharmacology of the commonly used agents.

● α agonists produce vasoconstriction. Cardiac α receptors have a very small positive inotropic effect.
● β1 agonists increase myocardial contractility and heart rate.
● β2 agonists produce peripheral vasodilatation (and bronchodilatation), increased myocardial contractility and reflex tachycardia.
● DA receptor agonism is dose-dependent. At low doses there is splanchnic dilatation, with improvements in renal, gut and liver blood flow. At higher doses, reuptake and produces vasoconstriction noradrenaline release.

This translates into the drug effects shown in Table 3.3.

TABLE 3.3 Drug effects		
Drug	**Receptor**	**Actions**
Adrenaline	β1 β2 α	↑ Heart rate & stroke volume (peripheral vasoconstriction)
Dobutamine	β1 (β2)	↑ Heart rate & stroke volume (peripheral vasodilatation)
Dopexamine	β2 DA	Peripheral & splanchnic vasodilatation (↑ heart rate)
Dopamine	DA	Increased renal perfusion*
Actions of dopamine dose dependant (see below).		

The choice of inotrope will therefore depend upon the clinical circumstances.

Adrenaline (0.1–0.5 μg/kg/min). At low doses the primary effect is increased CO whilst at higher doses there is additional potent vasoconstriction. It is useful in low output states associated with low peripheral vasomotor tone and low mean arterial pressure. Adrenaline is the drug of choice in an emergency and in hypotensive states when the overall haemodynamic status is not clear.

Dobutamine (1–20 µg/kg/min). Increases CO and causes a variable degree of peripheral vasodilatation. It is useful in low CO states when vasomotor tone and mean arterial pressure are reasonably maintained.

Dopexamine (1–5 µg/kg/min). At doses up to 1 µg/kg/min dopexamine has little inotropic activity and increases in cardiac output are mediated primarily by peripheral vasodilatation (reduced afterload) and reflex tachycardia. This results in improved blood flow primarily in the splanchnic and renal circulation. At doses above these, there is some intrinsic inotropic activity.

Dopexamine is useful in low cardiac output states when there is increased peripheral vasomotor tone and mean arterial blood pressure is maintained. In addition it may be used to promote renal – splanchnic blood flow. (See Oliguria, p. 120 and GIT failure p. 108.)

Dopamine (2.5–5 µg/kg/min). Dopamine acts on α, β and DA receptors and releases noradrenaline from adrenergic nerves. The actions of dopamine therefore vary depending on the dose.

At low doses, up to 5 µg/kg/min, the primary action is on DA receptors, resulting in increased splanchnic and renal perfusion. Dopamine may therefore be useful to help maintain renal blood flow and promote urine output. (See Oliguria p. 120.) At doses above 5 µg/kg/min dopamine vasoconstrictor and cardiac effects predominate. Do not use higher doses. If vasoconstrictor or cardiac inotrope doses are required use a more suitable alternative.

Selection of inotrope

Select the appropriate inotrope according to the patient's clinical condition. Generally start the lowest infusion rate possible to achieve the desired effect and continually reassess the response. Inotropes can behave unpredictably in the critically ill patient.

● Use adrenaline if low cardiac output is associated with low mean arterial blood pressure.
● Use dobutamine or dopexamine if low cardiac output is associated with adequate mean arterial blood pressure.
● Use dopamine only at low doses to promote renal perfusion.

OPTIMIZING PERFUSION PRESSURE

If despite adequate filling and best achievable cardiac output, the mean arterial pressure remains low, then vasoconstrictors should be used. The commonly available agents are:

● Phenylephrine (1–5 µg/kg/min).
● Noradrenaline (0.1–0.5 µg/kg/min).

Both drugs have direct action on α receptors and increase blood pressure by causing vasoconstriction. There is no appreciable direct effect on cardiac output. They are used to generate an adequate perfusion pressure for vital organs, in particular the brain, liver and kidneys.

Excessive use of vasoconstrictors may, however, be associated with a number of adverse effects. These include, increased afterload and reduced cardiac output, reduced renal blood flow, reduced splanchnic blood flow and impaired peripheral perfusion. Vasoconstrictors should, therefore, be used only in the lowest possible doses required to achieve the desired effect. In particular vasoconstrictors should only be titrated against the mean arterial blood pressure and not other derived variables such as systemic vascular resistance.

Warning! When interpreting the information gained from pulmonary artery catheters, you should remember that systemic vascular resistance is mathematically derived from CO and perfusion pressure, and is not a directly measured, independent variable.

Systemic Vascular Resistance = Perfusion Pressure × constant/Cardiac Output
$$SVR = (MAP–CVP) \times 80/CO$$

Therefore, vasoconstrictors should be titrated against blood pressure and not against the SVR.

RATIONAL USE OF INOTROPES AND VASOCONSTRICTORS

- Except in emergency, do not start inotropes or vasoconstrictors until adequate fluid loading has been achieved. Give only into central veins, using dedicated lines. Do not mix drugs.
- Use inotropes to increase CO.
- Use vasoconstrictors only when blood pressure remains low despite adequate fluid loading and best achievable CO.
- Dopamine (or dopexamine) may be used to promote renal blood flow.
- Continually reassess.

Following each change in therapy you should reassess the patient's haemodynamic status. In particular check filling status is still optimal and whether therapies have had the desired effects. When optimal haemodynamic status is apparently achieved, ensure oxygen delivery is adequate and consider markers of regional perfusion such as renal output.

No response to inotropes/vasoconstrictors

- Check that arterial and other monitoring lines are functioning correctly (check blood pressure manually) and that transducers are appropriately zeroed and at the correct level.

● Ensure that filling status is optimal. Inotropes and vasoconstrictors are of little value if the circulation is empty!

● Exclude mechanical causes of low CO and hypotension such as tension pneumothorax, pulmonary embolus and cardiac tamponade.

● Ensure that the appropriate inotrope or vasoconstrictor agent has been started. Check that the infusion is running at the correct rate. Note that if an infusion is started at a low rate it may take some time for the active drug to reach the end of the dead space in the infusion line.

● The myocardium responds poorly to inotropes in the presence of acidosis. Therefore if a significant acidosis is present (pH < 7.2) consider correcting this with sodium bicarbonate. (See Metabolic acidosis, p. 137.)

● Check the ionized calcium and consider giving additional calcium. (Never give calcium and sodium bicarbonate together down the same line!)

● If there is no improvement in haemodynamic status increase the infusion rate until an appropriate response is obtained. If there is still no response and particularly if the inotropes or vasoconstrictors have been in use for some time consider the possibility of tachyphylaxis and receptor down regulation. Start an alternative or additional agent.

● Consider the possibility of adrenocortical failure. This is very rare. (See Adrenal insuficiency, p. 142.)

Weaning inotropes and vasoconstrictors

As the patient's condition improves inotropes and vasoconstrictor agents can be gradually reduced. The procedure is in many ways similar to the above. Ensure optimal filling at all times and reduce drugs according to the results of haemodynamic monitoring. Where possible, reduce vasoconstrictors before inotropes.

COMMON PROBLEM: HYPOTENSION

(See Optimizing haemodynamic status above, p. 49.)

Assess the patient

● Is the blood pressure adequate for the patient? A MAP of 60 mmHg is generally adequate but this will depend on the patient's normal blood pressure which will vary with age and premorbid state.

● Is there evidence of inadequate tissue oxygenation or organ perfusion (acidosis, oliguria, or altered conscious level)? If not, further treatment may not be necessary.

● Is there an obvious cause for hypotension, e.g. hypovolaemia (bleeding), myocardial failure, sepsis? This will guide specific treatment.

Optimize filling status

● Unless there is evidence of fluid overload or myocardial failure, give a fluid challenge to optimize cardiac filling, even if measured CVP is apparently adequate, (e.g. 100–500 ml colloid). If there is no response (particularly if there is no rise in measured filling pressures) consider a further fluid bolus.

● If there is still no response establish invasive monitoring with a pulmonary artery catheter in order to measure PAOP and CO. (*See Practical procedures, p. 243.*)

> **Warning! Faced with significant hypotension in the absence of information from a pulmonary artery catheter, start an adrenaline infusion. This has both inotrope and vasoconstrictor actions and is the agent of choice in the first instance. It can be continued or replaced once invasive monitoring is established.**

Optimize cardiac output

● Give further fluid bolus if appropriate to increase PAOP and observe the change in CO. Titrate fluids to determine PAOP that gives optimum cardiac output.

● If CO remains low, add an inotrope. The choice will depend on the clinical condition of the patient. If the peripheral resistance is low adrenaline is useful as a first line.

Optimize perfusion pressure

● If mean arterial blood pressure remains low despite adequate filling pressure and cardiac output, add a vasoconstrictor to maintain diastolic blood pressure, e.g. noradrenaline. (See also Cardiogenic shock, p. 70 and Sepsis, p. 201.)

COMMON PROBLEM: HYPERTENSION

Although hypotension is more of a problem in intensive care, hypertension can also occur. This may be a manifestation of pre-existing essential hypertension, but is frequently secondary to other factors.

Causes of hypertension in ICU
● Preexisting hypertension/vascular disease
● Intracranial lesion
● Pain and anxiety
● Effects of exogenous catecholamines
● Hypervolaemia
● Hypoxia
● Hypercarbia
● Hypothermia

Management of hypertension

In intensive care short periods of hypertension, for example, during weaning from ventilation are not uncommon and do not generally result in any harm unless there is associated myocardial or vascular disease. Therefore:

- Do not overtreat hypertension.
- If using an arterial line check the blood pressure by sphygmomanometry. The readings sometimes disagree, in which case the non-invasive measurement may be the more accurate. (*See arterial cannulation, p. 227*)
- Ensure adequate analgesia and sedation.
- Ensure normal fluid status and blood gases.
- Reduce or stop inotropes and vasoconstrictors as appropriate.

Treatment will depend upon the absolute blood pressure, age and condition of the patient. The typical hypertensive patient is the elderly postoperative arteriopath with ischaemic heart disease. Treatment is generally only required if there is sustained diastolic blood pressure > 110 mmHg, systolic > 200 mmHg or associated myocardial ischaemia. If treatment is required consider:

- Nifedepine 10–20 mg sl. (Nifedepine capsules can be punctured with a needle and the contents given sublingually. This produces a gentle reduction in blood pressure within 20 min and can be repeated 6–8 hourly.)
- Hydrallazine 10 mg IV repeated as necessary.
- GTN infusion. Particularly if hypertensive episodes are associated with myocardial ischaemia or failure.
- Labetolol is used in small incremental boluses (5–10 mg) and by infusion.

 Warning! The use of β blockers to treat hypertension is best avoided as first line management in intensive care.

Young hypertensive patient

The young patient with unexplained sustained hypertension particularly if associated with end organ damage, for example, left ventricular hypertrophy, warrants further investigation. Consider other causes such as renal artery stenosis or endocrine such as phaeochromocytoma. (See Metabolic and endocrine, p. 143.)

DISTURBANCE OF CARDIAC RHYTHM

Disturbances in cardiac rhythm are common in the intensive care unit and this highlights the need for careful monitoring of all patients. Dysrhythmias may result from any underlying heart disease, e.g. ischaemic heart disease, cardiac myopathy or valve lesions.

Factors predisposing to dysrhythmia

- Pain & anxiety (inadequate analgesia and sedation)
- Increased catecholamine levels (endogenous or from inotrope infusions)
- Hypoxia
- Hypercarbia
- Endocrine abnormalities
- Electrolyte disturbance (hypokalaemia, hyperkalaemia, hypomagnesaemia)
- Hypovolaemia
- Pyrexia and myocardial effects of sepsis
- Drugs

Initially, ensure adequate oxygenation and ventilation together with correction of predisposing factors. Where there is no improvement or there is haemodynamic disturbance, definitive treatment is required.

Sinus tachycardia

This is a common problem and generally represents an appropriate response to factors listed above. Management is, therefore, correction of the underlying cause(s). For example, giving adequate sedation may unmask relative hypovolaemia requiring additional fluids.

 Warning! Do not give β blockers to control sinus tachycardia. This may result in decompensation.

Sinus bradycardia

Sinus bradycardia frequently reflects intrinsic disease of pacemaker tissue or conducting system. It may be precipitated by increased vagal tone, hypoxia (particularly in children) and the myocardial depressant effect of drugs. As heart rate falls initially CO is maintained by increases in SV but as heart rate falls further CO and blood pressure will fall. Junctional or ventricular escape rhythms may appear.

In the intensive care unit, if bradycardia occurs in association with significant hypotension then consider adrenaline. Give 50–100 µg (0.5–1 ml of 1: 10 000 adrenaline) boluses and titrate to effect (Fig. 3.3).

Supraventricular tachycardia (SVT)

SVT encompasses all forms of tachyarrhythmia originating above the ventricles. In practice it is useful to distinguish atrial fibrillation and atrial flutter from other forms of SVT. In SVT the QRS complexes are always narrow unless there is an associated conduction defect (Fig. 3.4).

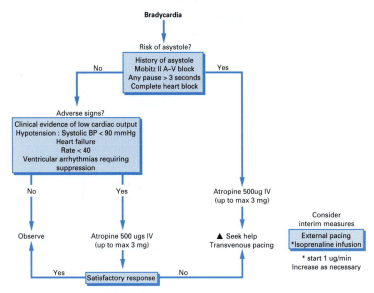

Fig. 3.3 Management of bradycardia. Doses based on adult of average body weight. In all cases give oxygen and establish IV access.

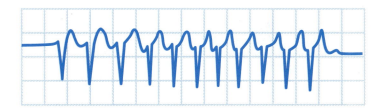

Fig. 3.4 Supraventricular tachycardia.

The management depends on the degree of haemodynamic disturbance.
Amiodarone may be the drug of choice for the treatment of SVT that is not associated with haemodynamic compromise (Fig. 3.5). Magnesium is also useful (see below).

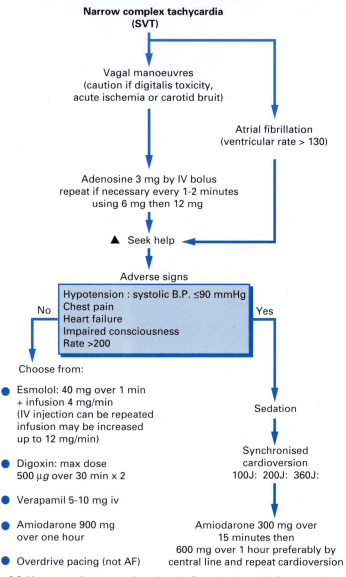

Fig. 3.5 Management of narrow complex tachycardia. Doses based on adult of average body weight. In all cases give oxygen and establish IV access. (Redrawn from Advanced Life Support Manual 2nd edn. 1994 Resuscitation Council, UK.)

Atrial fibrillation (AF)

This is the commonest dysrhythmia seen in intensive care (Fig. 3.6), particularly in the elderly patient with postoperative sepsis and inotrope dependency. Consider the underlying causes of dysrhythmia above. When sudden in onset, restoration of sinus rhythm (where possible) should be attempted. Treatment depends on the ventricular rate and the degree of associated haemodynamic disturbance. Sinus rhythm may return spontaneously as the underlying disease process resolves.

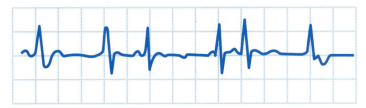

Fig. 3.6 Atrial fibrillation.

Use the SVT protocol above but note:

● For acute AF without haemodynamic compromise, amiodarone is more likely to restore sinus rhythm than digoxin. Amiodarone 300 mg over 30 minutes, followed by 900 mg over the next 24 hours. Larger doses are frequently required.
● Chronic AF may be associated with ischaemic heart disease or mitral valve disease. Restoration of sinus rhythm is unlikely and control of the ventricular rate is the main aim.

Digoxin is infused 0.5 mg IV over 30 minutes, followed by 0.25–0.5 mg after 2 hours if necessary. Once daily dose, thereafter, depending on response and levels.

There is increasing use of magnesium sulphate to treat supraventricular dysrhythmias. This is as effective as amiodarone in reverting AF to sinus rhythm. Typical dose is 10–20 mmol over 10 minutes followed by 50–100 mmol over 24 hours.

Atrial flutter

In atrial flutter (Fig. 3.7) the atrial rate is about 300 beats per minute and the P waves have a saw tooth appearance. The AV node cannot conduct all the P waves to the ventricle and there is often associated 2:1 AV block. Therefore, suspect if the ventricular rate is 150. At this rate use a 12 lead ECG to identify flutter waves.

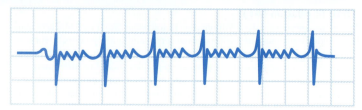

Fig. 3.7 Atrial flutter.

● Synchronized DC cardioversion (50J: 100J: 200J) is the treatment of choice.

DC cardioversion
Prior to 'elective' DC cardioversion, consider the need for anticoagulation (usually unnecessary except in chronic dysrhythmias). Check the patient is adequately sedated/anaesthetized. This may involve supplementing the sedation of a ventilated patient with a small (5–20 mg) dose of diazemuls. Awake patients require anaesthesia, usually with a cardiostable drug such as 0.1–0.2 mg/kg etomidate. Maintain oxygenation with 100% oxygen by facemask (before, during and after the anaesthetic). With the defibrillator in synchronized mode, the paddles are applied at the sternum and cardiac apex. Select the energy level and charge the paddles. Give an 'all clear' warning so that no-one is touching the patient when the shock is given. After delivery of the shock, several seconds may pass before monitors yield an ECG trace. If DC cardioversion fails, consider:

● Higher energy shock.
● Alternative paddle position (cardiac long axis, anteroposterior).
● Use of antiarrhythmic drug before repeat attempts.

Ventricular premature beats (VPBs)
VPBs occur normally in the general population and their significance is uncertain. They are more common in the presence of heart disease and may be increased by the effects of digoxin toxicity catecholamines and hypokalaemia. Asymptomatic unifocal VPB occurring less than 5 per minute are benign. Consider treatment if associated with poor haemodynamic state, multifocal, or occurring in runs of two or more.

● Correct hypoxia, hypercarbia, acidosis and hypokalaemia.
● Consider lignocaine 1 mg/kg followed by infusion 2 mg/min.
● Consider magnesium.

Broad complex tachycardia
Supra ventricular dysrhythmias may present as broad complex tachycardia if it is associated with aberrant conduction, for example, preexisting bundle branch block. Haemodynamic status depends largely on left ventricular function, so it is a poor guide to the underlying rhythm. Broad complex tachycardia should be assumed to be ventricular unless proved otherwise (Figs 3.8 and 3.9).

Broad complex tachycardia VT more likely if:
QRS very broad > 0.14 s
Evidence of AV dissociation
(capture beats or fusion beats)
Dominant first R wave in V1
Deep S wave V6
QRS direction same all V leads

Ventricular tachycardia (VT Fig. 3.8)

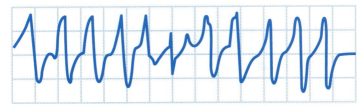

Fig. 3.8 Ventricular tachycardia.

Polymorphic ventricular tachycardia (Torsade de Pointes)

Torsades de pointes is a form of VT in which the complexes have a pointed shape, vary from beat to beat and the axis of the rhythm constantly changes. It is usually selflimiting but may give rise to VF. Hypokalaemia, prolonged QT interval, bradycardia and antiarrhythmic drugs may be causes.

● Give magnesium 10 mmol IV stat followed by 50 mmol infusion over 12 hours.
● β blockers.
● Seek expert help, consider overdrive pacing and DC cardioversion.

CONDUCTION DEFECTS

In addition to the dysrhythmias discussed above A-V conduction defects can result in haemodynamic compromise.

1st degree heart block
P–R interval >0.2 seconds (1 large square). This does not require treatment but is indicative of underlying heart disease, electrolyte disturbance or drug (digoxin) toxicity.

2nd degree heart block
This may be of 2 types.

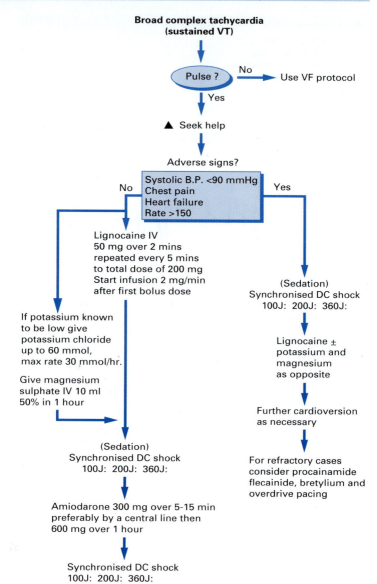

Fig. 3.9 Management of broad complex tachycardia. Doses based on adult of average body weight. In all cases give oxygen and establish IV access.

Mobitz type 1 (Wenkebach phenomenon). There is progressive lengthening of the P–R interval followed by a P wave which is not conducted to the ventricle and then repetition of the cycle. This is usually selflimiting and also does not require treatment.

Mobitz type 2. The P–R interval is constant but occasional P waves are not conducted to the ventricle. If high levels of block are present 2:1 or 3:1 block, etc. may develop. There is a significant risk that this will progress to complete heart block.

Complete heart block

No P waves are conducted to the ventricle. This may result in ventricular standstill (no CO!) or there may be an idioventricular escape rhythm. In this case there is no discernible relationship between the P waves and QRS complexes on the ECG.

1st and 2nd degree heart block does not require treatment. However, any episode of heart block which is symptomatic requires treatment.

- See bradycardia algorithm above.
- Consider pacing – external or temporary pacing wire.

Indications for temporary pacing wire

Symptomatic bradycardia unresponsive to treatment (See *algorithm*)
Mobitz type 2 heart block
Complete heart block
RBBB + left anterior or posterior hemiblock in association with prolonged PR interval*
*Relative indication.

MYOCARDIAL ISCHAEMIA

Ischaemic heart disease (IHD) is extremely common and ranges from the asymptomatic, through stable angina to crescendo angina and myocardial infarction.

Many patients admitted to intensive care will already be on a number of cardiovascular medications and these should be reviewed in the light of the patient's condition. Where appropriate, existing drug therapy should be continued, however, many oral cardiac drugs have no parenteral preparation. In practice it is common to stop such medication in the acute phase of a critical illness and reintroduce it as the patient's condition improves.

- Oral nitrates can be replaced with GTN patches (5–10 mg every 24 hours) or GTN infusion.
- Warfarin (for prosthetic valves or chronic AF) should be replaced by heparin infusion and the APTT monitored. The required level will depend upon the indication for coagulation.

- Diuretics may be continued in equivalent doses IV.
- Ca^{2+} channel blockers, β blockers and ACE inhibitors are usually withheld.

Most patients in the ICU are unable to indicate the onset of ischaemic chest pain because of the effects of sedation and ventilation. However, changes in ECG monitoring such as ST depression and deteriorating myocardial performance such as reduced CO may indicate ischaemia. The management will depend upon the apparent degree of ischaemia and associated haemodynamic disturbance.

Simple angina/ST depression

- Give oxygen.
- Correct precipitating factors such as tachycardia/hypertension or hypotension.
- Administer GTN either sublingually or as oral spray. Consider GTN infusion.
- Give analgesia if required. Usually bolus of morphine or diamorphine IV.

Unstable angina/increasing ST depression (crescendo angina)

If angina and ST depression do not settle or become more severe, myocardial infarction may be imminent. The commonest mechanism of infarction is rupture of a soft atheromatous plaque and subsequent occlusive thrombus formation within the coronary artery. Management is based at preventing this. In addition to the above:

- Consider β blocker (atenolol 100 mg daily) if there are no contraindications (bradycardia, hypotension, heart failure, asthma).
- Start GTN infusion to reduce preload and reduce myocardial work.
1–2 mg/hour. Titrate to response.
- Start heparin infusion 24 000 unit over 24 hours.
- Give aspirin 150 mg oral daily (contraindications GI bleed, asthma, renal impairment).

ACUTE MYOCARDIAL INFARCTION

The diagnosis of myocardial infarction is made on the basis of a characteristic history of chest pain, ECG evidence and retrospective interpretation of cardiac enzymes.

ECG changes

The typical ECG changes accompanying acute myocardial infarction are:

- ST segment elevation > 1 mm in precordial leads or 2 mm in limb leads which persists for more than 24 hours. Usually returns to normal within 2 weeks. (Persistent ST elevation at 1 month suggests development of left ventricular aneurysm).
- Reciprocal ST segment depression in the opposite leads.
- Development of new Q waves greater than 25% of the 'R' wave and 0.04 sec duration.
- T wave inversion. (This is not diagnostic by itself.)

The location of these changes on the ECG identify the region of the infarction (see Table 3.4).

TABLE 3.4 Location of changes on ECG	
Area of infarction	**ECG leads:**
Inferior	AF, II & III
Anteroseptal	VI–V4
Anterior	V3–V4
Anterolateral	V3–V6

Enzyme changes

Typical patterns of enzyme changes following myocardial infarction are shown in Figure 3.10 and Table 3.5.

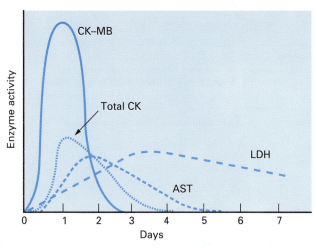

Fig. 3.10 Cardiac enzymes pattern of change.

TABLE 3.5 Patterns of enzyme changes		
Enzyme	**Peak**	**Duration**
Creatinine kinase (CK–MB)	12–24 hours	1.5–3 days
Total Creatinine kinase	18–30 hours	2–5 days
Aspartate transaminase (AST)	20–30 hours	2–6 days
Lactate dehydrogenase (LDH)	30–48 hours	5–14 days

CK–MB

This is the most useful diagnostic enzyme test. Creatinine phosphokinase (CK) is released from all damaged muscle, whereas CK–MB is specific to heart muscle. If the total CK is raised and the ratio of CK–MB to CK is greater than 6–8% then myocardial infarction is highly likely. This is particularly useful in the context of postoperative myocardial infarction when total CK, AST and LDH may all be raised for other reasons.

Patients may be admitted to intensive care following a myocardial infarction or may suffer an infarction during their treatment in the intensive care. In this case, the history of classic chest pain is not always available and treatment may have to be commenced on the basis of ECG changes and the accompanying clinical picture. This may include the sudden development of hypotension, cardiac failure (3rd or 4th heart sound), pericardial rub and mild pyrexia. If myocardial infarction is suspected perform serial ECG and cardiac enzyme studies for three days.

Management

Management is similar to crescendo angina above.

- Oxygen.
- Analgesia.
- Consider β blocker, e.g. atenolol 100 mg daily, if there are no contraindications (bradycardia, hypotension, heart failure, asthma).
- Consider GTN infusion to reduce preload and reduce myocardial work. 1–2 mg/hour. Titrate to response.
- Consider thrombolysis. Steptokinase 1.5 million units in 100–200 ml 0.9% saline IV over 1 hour.

Thrombolysis aims to limit the size of myocardial infarction by dissolving coronary artery thrombus and reperfusing the myocardium. This is only indicated if there is irrefutable ECG evidence of acute infarction. It should then be started as soon as possible and preferably within 6 hours of the onset of chest pain unless there are contraindications.

Contraindications to thrombolysis

Recent surgery
Intracranial pathology, e.g. previous CVA
Previous GI haemorrhage
Bleeding from any site
Allergy to streptokinase
Prolonged external cardiac massage

Most patients who develop myocardial infarction in the ICU will have some contraindication to thrombolysis. If thrombolysis is contraindicated, consider starting a heparin infusion.

- Heparin infusion 24 000 unit over 24 hours.
- Give aspirin 150 mg oral daily (contraindications GI bleed, asthma, renal impairment).
- Bradycardia, heart block and dysrhythmias are common following myocardial infarction.

Postoperative myocardial infarction

Postoperative myocardial infarction is associated with a high mortality (>50%). Patients should be managed in the ICU as above. Thrombolytic therapy is often contraindicated because of the risk of bleeding from the surgical site.

Early consultation with the cardiologists is advisable and consideration given to the possibility of acute angiography with angioplasty or acute coronary artery bypass grafting.

CARDIAC FAILURE

Heart failure is common and represents an inability of the heart to maintain sufficient CO despite adequate filling. The clinical picture may range from mild peripheral oedema and shortness of breath to florid pulmonary oedema and hypotension. The principles of management are the same:

- Given oxygen. Consider CPAP by face mask or non-invasive ventilation.
- Institute invasive monitoring as necessary. Arterial line and pulmonary artery catheter.
- Optimize preload. Consider the use of diuretics and GTN infusion to reduce both preload and afterload.
- Add an inotrope.
- ACE inhibitors have been shown to improve survival in cardiac failure. Consider the use of these as early as possible. (These drugs may cause severe first dose hypotension and should be introduced gradually. Also consider carefully in renal impairment.)

Right heart failure and pulmonary hypertension

Mitral valve disease and chronic pulmonary disease may result in pulmonary hypertension and subsequent right heart failure. This is a very difficult condition to manage. When pulmonary artery and right ventricular pressures are high, systemic pressure falls and perfusion of the right ventricle is impaired. This results in worsening right ventricular performance and rapid deterioration.

- Avoid drugs that lower systemic pressure. (Vasoconstrictors may be necessary to maintain systemic blood pressure and right ventricular perfusion.)
- Optimal filling of the right ventricle is vital. This may require the use of specialist monitoring such as right heart ejection fraction pulmonary artery catheters, which can directly estimate right ventricular end diastolic volume.
- Inotropes may improve right ventricular contractility.

● Prostacycline may be used to reduce pulmonary artery pressure and thus reduce right ventricular afterload. In practice this is not selective and may also reduce systemic blood pressure.

● Nitric oxide may be useful particularly when pulmonary hypertension is secondary to hypoxic pulmonary vasoconstriction associated with primary lung disease. (See: ARDS p. 98.)

CARDIOGENIC SHOCK

This is the failure to adequately perfuse tissue as a result of poor cardiac function. It is characterized by high cardiac filling pressures, low cardiac output and increased systemic vascular resistance. This is associated with a very high mortality. The main aim is to restore oxygen delivery to tissues by increasing CO.

● Ventilate with 100% oxygen and correct any dysrhythmias (non-invasive ventilation may be appropriate).

● Establish invasive monitoring with arterial pressure and pulmonary artery catheter.

● Optimize filling pressure. Cardiogenic shock is generally associated with a high PAOP and pulmonary oedema. Consider diuretics to remove fluid. Vasodilators such as GTN may reduce preload if the blood pressure is adequate.

● Rationalize inotropes. In the first instance adrenaline infusion is the inotrope of choice. This will increase CO and maintain some degree of peripheral vasoconstriction. Once invasive monitoring is established inodilator drugs such as dopexamine and dobutamine may be more appropriate.

● If CO fails to improve, consider enoximone. This is a phosphodiesterase inhibitor, (PDE-III) which acts at an intracellular level, effectively bypassing the β receptors. It is an inodilator, and causes both an increase in CO and peripheral vasodilatation. It may be associated with a marked fall in blood pressure. Do not give loading doses, start infusion at a low level and increase according to response. Hypotension may require concomitant use of a vasoconstrictor such as noradrenaline to maintain adequate diastolic pressure.

● Where there is no improvement with these measures, consider intraaortic balloon counter pulsation. The balloon is inserted via a femoral artery and inflates in the aorta during diastole to maintain diastolic perfusion of the myocardium.

CARDIAC ARREST

Most deaths in the ICU are expected and sudden unexpected cardiac arrest is actually infrequent. If patients arrest despite optimal intensive care management, unless the problem is one of transient ventricular dysrhythmia, it is unlikely that the outcome will be favourable. You should follow the algorithms published by the Resuscitation Council (UK).

Ventricular fibrillation (VF)/pulseless ventricular tachycardia

The chances of a successful outcome from VF is best if defibrillation is achieved within 90 seconds of onset and decrease with time thereafter. In a witnessed arrest a single precordial thump may terminate fibrillation after which the application of defibrillating DC shock should not be delayed (Fig. 3.11).

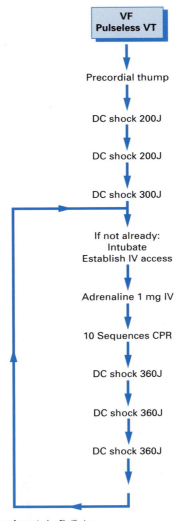

Fig. 3.11 Management of ventricular fibrillation.

Asystole

Chances of recovery from asystolic arrest are poor. Be sure that the diagnosis is correct. Check that the ECG leads are correctly attached and that the gain on the monitor is maximal. If VF cannot be excluded, then management commences as for VF (Fig. 3.12).

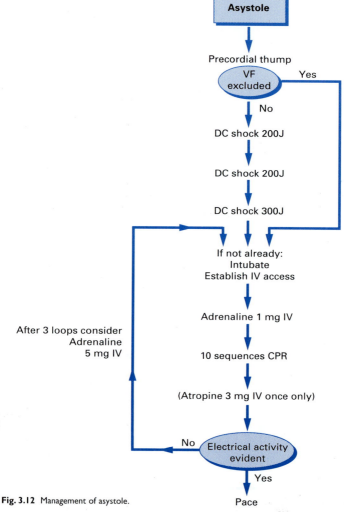

Fig. 3.12 Management of asystole.

Electromechanical dissociation

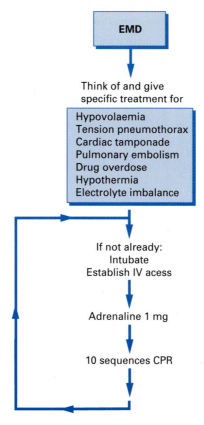

EMD

Think of and give
specific treatment for

Hypovolaemia
Tension pneumothorax
Cardiac tamponade
Pulmonary embolism
Drug overdose
Hypothermia
Electrolyte imbalance

If not already:
Intubate
Establish IV acess

Adrenaline 1 mg

10 sequences CPR

Fig. 3.13 Management of electromechanical dissociation.

Management of patients following cardiac arrest

Patients who are resuscitated from cardiac arrest outside the ICU frequently
require admission to intensive care. The management of these patients depends
upon the underlying clinical condition, the type of arrest and the adequacy of
initial resuscitation measures. The main difficulty is determining the extent
and nature of neurological injury resulting from the period of hypoxia. It is
very difficult to make any assessment of this in the first 24–48 hours and in
particular apparently fixed and dilated pupils are an unreliable sign. Most
patients, therefore, will require a period of stabilization and assessment.

- Institute positive pressure ventilation according to arterial blood gases.
- Optimize haemodynamic status.
- Correct acidosis and electrolyte abnormalities.
- Treat any underlying conditions appropriately.

It is reasonable to avoid sedation initially until the neurological condition improves sufficiently either to warrant sedation or to make weaning and extubation feasible. If the patient's neurological condition fails to improve over 48 hours then the outcome is likely to be poor. (See Hypoxic brain injury, p. 180.)

CHAPTER 4

RESPIRATORY SYSTEM

DEFINITION OF RESPIRATORY FAILURE

Respiratory failure occurs when pulmonary gas exchange becomes sufficiently impaired such that normal arterial blood gas tensions are no longer maintained, and hypoxaemia is present with or without hypercapnia. Two patterns are described:

Type 1 (hypoxic) respiratory failure

$$Pa_{O_2} < 8 \text{ kPa with normal or low } Pa_{CO_2}$$

Type 1 respiratory failure is caused by disease processes which directly affect alveolar function, e.g. fibrosing alveolitis, pneumonia, pulmonary oedema, and adult respiratory distress syndrome. (ARDS).

Type 2 (hypercapnic) respiratory failure

$$Pa_{O_2} < 8 \text{ kPa and } Pa_{CO_2} > 8 \text{ kPa}$$

Type 2 respiratory failure is caused by failure of alveolar ventilation. It occurs most commonly in association with chronic obstructive airways disease (COAD) but may be caused by reduced respiratory drive, airway impairment, neuromuscular conditions and chest wall deformity.

Warning! These definitions are somewhat theoretical, since any patient with type 1 hypoxic respiratory failure will eventually become exhausted, develop alveolar hypoventilation and then retain carbon dioxide.

These definitions relate to patients breathing air at normal atmospheric pressure. When interpreting blood gases the inspired oxygen concentration (Fi_{O_2}) must be known. Clearly a patient who is already receiving significant oxygen therapy and still has poor Pa_{O_2} is considerably worse than a patient with the same Pa_{O_2} on air.

INTERPRETATION OF BLOOD GASES

The ability to interpret blood gases is fundamental to the management of all patients in intensive care and not just those with respiratory failure. Arterial samples are drawn into a heparinized syringe. Ensure that any liquid heparin is completely expelled from the syringe before use, as this will contaminate the sample and affect the results. Arterial blood is obtained either by direct puncture of an artery or from an indwelling arterial line. (See Practical procedures, Arterial cannulation p. 227.)

Most ICUs now have a blood gas analyzer. These are expensive to maintain and repair. If you do not know how to use it ask for help. Normal blood gas values are as shown in Table 4.1.

TABLE 4.1 Blood gas values

pH	7.35–7.45
Pao_2	13 kPa
$Paco_2$	5.3 kPa
St Hco_3	22–25 mmol/l
Base excess or deficit	−2 to +2 mmol/l

When interpreting blood gases from a patient use the following system:

● What is the inspired oxygen concentration? Look at the Pao_2. Is the patient hypoxic? What is the A–a gradient? (See APACHE scoring: calculating A–a gradient, p. 40.)

● Look at the $Paco_2$. Is it low, normal or high?

● Look at the pH. Is the patient acidotic (pH < 7.34) or alkalotic (pH < 7.45)?

If the patient has a disturbance of acid base balance then it is necessary to examine the blood gas further to determine the cause.

● Look again at the $Paco_2$. Is the $Paco_2$ consistent with the change in pH, i.e. if the patient is acidotic is the $Paco_2$ raised? If the patient is alkalotic is the $Paco_2$ low? If so the primary abnormality is respiratory.

● If the $Paco_2$ is normal or does not explain the abnormality in pH, look at the base deficit/base excess.

The base deficit/base excess is a calculation of how much base (e.g. bicarbonate) needs to be added to or taken away to normalize the pH of the sample. For example, in a metabolic acidosis, bicarbonate needs to be added to correct the pH because there is insufficient base present, i.e. there is a base deficit (< − 2 mmol/l). In metabolic alkalosis, bicarbonate needs to be taken away to correct the pH, because there is too much base present., i.e. there is a base excess (> + 2 mmol/l).

● If the base deficit/base excess is consistent with the abnormality in pH then the primary abnormality is metabolic.

● If both the Pco_2 and the base excess/base deficit are altered in a way that is consistent with the abnormality in pH then a mixed picture is present.

A number of patterns of disturbance of acid base balance can be recognized.

Respiratory acidosis

Hypoventilation from any cause, results in accumulation of CO_2, and respiratory acidosis. Over time, the bicarbonate concentration may rise (base excess) in an attempt to balance this and a compensated respiratory acidosis in which the pH is nearly normal may result.

Respiratory alkalosis

Hyperventilation may occur due to the effects of mechanical ventilation, or in response to hypoxaemia, drugs and injury to the central nervous system. This results in a lowering of the $Paco_2$ and a respiratory alkalosis. Bicarbonate concentration may fall (base deficit) in an attempt to compensate.

Metabolic acidosis

There are a number of causes of metabolic acidosis, resulting from the accumulation of organic acids, or the loss of bicarbonate buffer. Bicarbonate concentration is low (there is a base deficit). If the patient is breathing spontaneously, compensatory hyperventilation may result in a low $Pa\text{CO}_2$. (See Metabolic acidosis p. 137.)

Metabolic alkalosis

This is relatively uncommon and may result from the loss of acid, for example, from excessive vomiting or nasogastric drainage, or from excessive administration of alkali. Other causes include hypokalaemia, diuretics and liver failure. The bicarbonate concentration is raised + base excess) and the patient may hypoventilate in an attempt to compensate, resulting in a raised $Pa\text{CO}_2$. (See Metabolic alkalosis p. 139.)

ASSESSMENT OF A PATIENT WITH RESPIRATORY FAILURE

Causes of respiratory failure

Loss of respiratory drive
CVA/brain injury
Metabolic disturbance
Drugs
Neuromuscular disease
Spinal cord injury & disease
Phrenic nerve injury
Guillain–Barré/myasthenia
Neuromyopathy
Airway obstruction (upper & lower)
Foreign body
Tumour
Infection
Sleep apnoea
Pulmonary pathology
Asthma
Pneumonia
COAD
Chronic fibrosing conditions
ARDS
Chest wall deformity
Trauma
Thoracoplasty
Scoliosis

Blood gases are only one indicator of respiratory function. Primary assessment of a patient with respiratory failure is clinical.

- Can the patient talk; is he lucid? Take a history. If the patient is too short of breath to talk, history is from the notes, staff or relatives. Try to obtain some idea of the patient's normal respiratory reserve. How far can he/she walk? Is he/she chair bound or oxygen dependent?
- Look at the patient. Is he/she making adequate respiratory effort, using accessory muscles of respiration, or is respiratory effort minimal? Is he/she exhausted?
- Examine the patient – especially the cardiovascular and respiratory systems. Bear in mind the cause of respiratory failure. Note:
  — Pulse, BP (paradox?), JVP, heart sounds, peripheral oedema. Is there any evidence of cardiac failure or of dehydration?
  — Tachypnoea or hypopnoea, tracheal shift, percussion, bilateral air entry. Presence of crackles or wheeze. Is there any evidence of obstruction, collapse or consolidation, bronchospasm, pleural effusion?
- If there is wheeze, peak flow measurement may help to document severity but is often unrecordable in the critically ill.
- Look at CXR, blood gases and other available investigations.

MANAGEMENT OF RESPIRATORY FAILURE

 Warning! If the patient is in extremis due to respiratory failure then immediate action is required. Support respiration with a bag and mask using 100% oxygen. Intubate and continue positive pressure ventilation. Beware of cardiovascular collapse. (See Practical procedures: Intubation p. 247.)

- Hypoxia is the main concern and should be corrected. Give oxygen via a face mask, preferably by a high-flow, humidified system. If there is evidence of chronic CO_2 retention, give controlled oxygen therapy via a Venturi system. (See COAD p. 96.)
- Bronchodilators. If there is wheeze, nebulized bronchodilators may help. In more severe cases consider aminophylline infusion. (See Asthma p. 94.)
- Physiotherapy may help clear secretions and re-expand areas of collapse.
- Antibiotic therapy is best directed on the basis of Gram stains of sputum and on subsequent culture results. Seek microbiological advice. In the first instance broad-spectrum cover, e.g. with a cephalosporin is probably appropriate. Erythromycin may be added if there is a possibility of an atypical chest infection. (See Pneumonia p. 88.)
- Diuretics. If there is evidence of congestive cardiac failure and pulmonary oedema, then diuretics may help. Frusemide 40 mg or bumetanide 1–2 mg.

Continually reassess response to treatment. If there is no improvement or if the patient's condition worsens, intubation and ventilation may become necessary.

Indications for intervention
Exhaustion
Tachycardia/bradycardia
Hypotension
Increasing respiratory rate
Reduced conscious level
Falling PaO_2 despite oxygen therapy
Rising $PaCO_2$ despite therapy

● If the patient is gradually becoming exhausted and their clinical condition deteriorating, do not wait until they are moribund. Institute ventilation.

Role of non-invasive ventilation

The use of non-invasive forms of ventilation to manage patients with chronic respiratory failure is now well established. There is also increasing use of this form of treatment to manage patients with acute episodes of respiratory failure, particularly those with acute exacerbations of COAD. Pressure support ventilation or biphasic positive pressure ventilation can be provided by means of a tightly fitting face mask or nasal mask, which patients can remove intermittently to eat and drink. This is better tolerated by patients than endotracheal intubation and conventional ventilation and avoids many of the complications. Some patient groups may have improved outcome with non-invasive ventilation compared with conventional intermittent positive pressure ventilation (IPPV). Should a patient's condition fail to improve, conventional ventilation may still be required.

PRINCIPLES OF ARTIFICIAL VENTILATION

Most intensive care ventilators are now highly sophisticated, computer-controlled machines with complicated interfaces, a large number of different ventilatory modes, and inbuilt monitoring and alarm systems. Most complex modes are used for weaning. To date there is little evidence for their efficacy. They do, however, avoid the need for repeated changes of breathing circuit. Detailed description and discussion are beyond the scope of this book. Before using a ventilator you should familiarize yourself with it. If you have any difficulties seek senior advice.

Controlled mandatory ventilation (CMV)

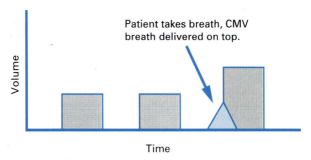

Fig. 4.1 Controlled mandatory ventilation.

This is the simplest form of ventilation in which the patient is ventilated at a preset tidal volume and rate (for example, Vt 800 ml × rate 12 breaths min). This is suitable for patients who are heavily sedated and or paralysed and who are making no respiratory effort. It is not suitable for patients who are attempting spontaneous breaths. Ventilator valves may be closed during attempted inspiration or expiration. The ventilator may deliver a breath immediately on top of the patient's own breath, or as the patient tries to breath out. This is uncomfortable and distressing, and may result in trauma to the lungs (see below).

Synchronized intermittent mandatory ventilation (SIMV)

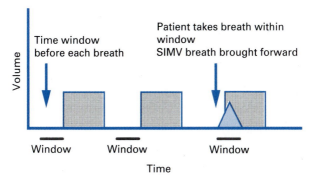

Fig. 4.2 Synchronized intermittent mandatory ventilation.

With this form of ventilation, tidal volume and rate are preset. Immediately before each breath there is a small time window during which the ventilator can recognize a spontaneous breath and responds by delivering the SIMV breath early. This prevents some of the problems that occur with CMV and is more comfortable for the patient. This form of ventilation is suitable for almost all patients in the ICU with the exception of those with severe acute lung injury.

Pressure control ventilation

Pressure control ventilation may be used both to reduce barotrauma and provide more effective ventilation to patients with non-compliant lungs. Respiratory rate is set. Instead of tidal volume, peak inspiratory pressure is set. When the ventilator delivers a breath, gas flows until the preset inspiratory pressure is achieved. Airway pressure is maintained for the duration of the breath. In this way tidal volume depends upon lung compliance. As the patient's condition improves and lung compliance increases, the tidal volume achieved for the same inspiratory pressure will increase. Hence pressure control can be reduced.

It is important with pressure control ventilation to understand the relationship between rate and inspiratory: expiratory ratio (I:E ratio). Rate determines the total time period for each breath (60 seconds divided by rate = duration in seconds for each breath.) The I:E ratio then determines how time is apportioned between inspiration and expiration.
For example.

> If respiratory rate 12
> Total time for breath 60/12 seconds = 5 seconds
> if I:E ratio 1:2 then
> Inspiratory time ≈ 1.6 seconds   Expiratory time ≈ 3.3 seconds

When the rate is reduced while I:E ratio is fixed, inspiratory time becomes progressively longer, effectively holding the patient in sustained inspiration. To avoid this the inspiratory time can be fixed (for example, 1.6 seconds) so that as the respiratory rate is changed it is only the length of expiration which alters.

Pressure support/assisted spontaneous breathing (ASB)

As patients improve they are weaned from artificial ventilation and take more breaths for themselves. Breathing through a ventilator can be difficult because respiratory muscles may be weak and ventilator circuits provide significant resistance to breathing. These problems can be minimized by the provision of pressure support. The ventilator senses a spontaneous breath and augments it by addition of positive pressure. This reduces the work of breathing for the patient and helps to augment the tidal volume that would otherwise have been achieved.

● Set the pressure support at 15–20 cm H_2O initially. This can be reduced as the patient's condition improves. (It is best not to remove pressure support completely, because of the resistance of the ventilator). (See Weaning from artificial ventilation p. 87.)

Positive end expiratory pressure (PEEP)

Intubation and artificial ventilation result in changes in functional residual capacity (FRC) of the lung and alterations in the distribution of ventilation. This in turn causes small airways particularly in dependant lung zones to collapse and results in increasing shunt and worsening blood gases. To prevent this +5 to +10 cm H_2O of PEEP can be used to help maintain FRC and alveolar recruitment. Disadvantages of PEEP include reduced venous return to the heart and a subsequent reduction in CO and blood pressure. Unnecessarily high levels of PEEP are therefore, best avoided. PEEP is relatively contraindicated in asthmatics, and in chronic emphysema.

Continuous positive airway pressure (CPAP)

CPAP is a system for spontaneously breathing patients which is analogous to PEEP in ventilated patients. It may be provided either through a tight-fitting face-mask or via connection to an endotracheal/tracheostomy tube. A high gas flow (which must be greater than the patient's peak inspiratory flow rate) is generated in the breathing system. A valve on the expiratory port ensures that pressure in the system, and patient's airways, never falls below the set level. This is usually +5 to +10 cm H_2O. Relative disadvantages of CPAP include noise and problems with humidification.

Setting up a ventilator

In addition to setting the mode of ventilation, tidal volume and rate, a number of other variables need to be determined. Table 4.2 is a guide to the initial typical ventilator setting for an average adult. These will need to be altered in response to blood gases and changes in the patient's condition.

TABLE 4.2 Typical ventilator settings

Parameter	Setting
Mode ventilation	SIMV
Rate	8–14
Tidal volume (Vt)	700–800 ml (7–10 ml/kg)
Minute volume (MV)	5–8 litres/min (100 ml/kg/min)
Pressure support	15–20 cm H_2O
PEEP	5–7.5 cm H_2O
FiO_2	0.5–0.6 (depends on oxygenation)
I:E ratio	1:2

Monitoring ventilation

In addition to clinical progress and blood gases, ventilator function should be continuously monitored. Current intensive care ventilators have a large number of built-in monitors and alarms which do this, although you may have to set values for some of these. In particular you should note:

- Inspired oxygen concentration.
- Tidal volume and minute volume delivered and expired. A discrepancy between the two indicates a leak in the circuit.
- Peak airway pressure. If the peak airway pressure does not reach a predetermined value, the breathing circuit may have become disconnected. If the peak pressure is too high this may indicate obstruction of the airway, breathing circuit, or poor compliance. The patient may be at risk of barotrauma.
- Spontaneous effort. Many ventilators are able to record and measure any spontaneous contribution the patient makes to the minute volume.

Care of the ventilated patient

This encompasses many elements discussed earlier including provision of adequate analgesia, sedation, and psychological support. In addition, a number of other factors are important.

- Humidification. Some form of humidification is essential in every case. Adequate humidification prevents drying of secretions. This is generally provided by a heated water bath on the inspiratory limb of the ventilator circuit.
- Physiotherapy and tracheal suction.

The presence of an endotracheal tube and the effects of analgesia and sedation impair the ability to cough and clear secretions. Regular physiotherapy and suction of the airway is essential to prevent accumulation of secretions.

COMPLICATIONS OF IPPV

There are many complications of artificial ventilation. These include the following.

- Risks associated with endotracheal intubation, including inability to intubate, and dislodgement or blockage of the endotracheal tube. Prolonged intubation may be associated with damage to the larynx (particularly the vocal cords) and trachea. Traditionally tracheostomy was performed at about 14 days but many units now perform percutaneous tracheostomy earlier. (See Practical procedures: tracheostomy p. 251.)
- The drying effect of gases and impaired cough lead to retention of secretions and increases the likelihood of chest infection.
- Problems associated with the need for anaesthesia and or sedation and, in particular, the cardiovascular depressant effects of drugs. These drugs may cause gastric stasis and may delay the recovery. (See Sedation and analgesia p. 24.)
- Haemodynamic effects of IPPV and PEEP include reduced venous return, reduced CO and reduced blood pressure. In turn this reduces gut/renal blood flow and function.

● Barotrauma. The effects of high pressures applied to the airway can result in damage to the delicate tissues of the lung. This may be manifest as pneumothorax, pneumopericardium, subcutaneous surgical emphysema, interstitial emphysema and even air embolism. Where possible peak pressure should not be allowed to exceed 30–40 cm H_2O. If pressures above this are required consider the underlying cause and the need for pressure controlled ventilation and 'permissive hypercapnia'. (See ARDS p. 98.)

COMMON PROBLEM: POOR OXYGENATION

Gradual deterioration in oxygenation may represent continuing development of the pathophysiological process, whilst more sudden deterioration may represent the onset of a new problem or complication.

● Check the ventilator settings, Fio_2 and PEEP.
● Check the position of the endotracheal tube. Are both sides of the chest being ventilated equally? Are there any new clinical signs? Particularly, evidence of new collapse, pulmonary oedema and effusions, or pneumothorax. Obtain chest X-ray. (Effusions/pneumothoraces may be better demonstrated on erect or semi-erect films.)
● Treat any findings as appropriate. Increase Fio_2. Consider increasing PEEP, tidal volume, and altering the I:E ratio (increase the inspiratory time). Consider pressure control ventilation, or more sophisticated manoeuvres.
● Consider permissive hypoxaemia where aggressive ventilation is more likely than poor oxygenation to result in harm. Pao_2 above 8 kPa and Sao_2 above 88% are safe. (See ARDS, p. 98.)

COMMON PROBLEM: HYPERCAPNIA

Hypercapnia generally results from inadequate ventilator settings and is simply resolved. It may be associated with complications of ventilation which result in reduced compliance particularly pneumothorax. Occasionally it may result from hypermetabolic states in which there is increased CO_2 production.

● Check ventilator settings, tidal volume and rate. Ensure that dead space in the ventilator circuit is minimal.
● Check the position of the endotracheal tube. Are both sides of the chest being ventilated equally? Are there any new clinical signs? Particularly, evidence of pneumothorax. Get a chest X-ray if there is any doubt.
● Treat any findings as appropriate. Increase rate and/or tidal volume.
● Consider permissive hypercapnia: sometimes an elevated $Paco_2$ is appropriate, either because lung pathophysiology makes reduction difficult/hazardous, or because the patient's habitual $Paco_2$ is elevated. Remember head-injured patients and those at risk of raised intracranial pressure may be harmed by an elevated $Paco_2$.

COMMON PROBLEM: INCREASED AIRWAY PRESSURES

Increases in airway pressure generally indicate a significant problem and should be dealt with promptly, both to resolve the underlying cause and to prevent injury from barotrauma.

● Check patient. Is there partial or complete obstruction of the endotracheal tube or major airway? Suction may clear this. If in doubt, change the endotracheal tube.
● Are there any new clinical signs? Is there evidence of bronchospasm or pneumothorax? Treat any findings as appropriate. This may require physiotherapy and suction, improved humidification, nebulized bronchodilators.
● Check ventilator settings. Are tidal volume, I:E ratio, and inspiratory flow rate appropriate?
● If there is no evidence of an acute problem and airway pressures are rising due to reduced lung compliance or underlying pathophysiology, consider pressure control or alternative modes of ventilation.

ALTERNATIVE MODES OF VENTILATION

In patients with low pulmonary compliance, conventional IPPV can result in high airway pressures, barotrauma and haemodynamic disturbance. High frequency ventilation has been tried as a means of reducing transpulmonary pressure, while providing adequate gas exchange. In most cases the tidal volume generated is less than anatomical dead space, and the exact mechanisms by which gas exchange is maintained are poorly understood. If you are considering these alternative modes of ventilation seek senior advice.

1. High frequency oscillation
A piston oscillates a diaphragm across the open airway resulting in a sinusoidal flow pattern with I:E ratio 1:1. This is unique in that both inspiration and expiration are active. Airway pressure oscillates gently around a mean. Increasing the mean airway pressure recruits more alveoli and improves oxygenation. CO_2 clearance is controlled by altering the rate. Clearance of secretions is improved. This type of ventilation is currently used primarily in neonatal and paediatric intensive care.

2. Jet ventilation
Pulses of gas are delivered at high pressure through a cannula placed in a T-piece or via a special endotracheal tube. The driving pressure and rate can be set. The jet of gas entrains air/oxygen from an open circuit. Tidal volume generated is generally of the order of 70–170 ml, and expiration is passive. Typical settings are shown in Table 4.3.

TABLE 4.3 Typical settings for jet ventilation

FiO_2	0.6–1.0
Driving pressure	1.5–3 atmospheres
	(150–300 kPa)
Frequency	60–200
I:E Ratio	1:1

There are two main roles for jet ventilation.

● Management of bronchopleural fistulae. During conventional ventilation most of the tidal volume may be lost through the fistula making effective ventilation of the patient impossible. Jet ventilation is claimed to reduce transpulmonary pressures thus reducing the leak.

● Aid to weaning. Patients can comfortably breathe over jet ventilation. As the patient's condition improves, driving pressure is reduced and frequency increased.

The technique can be noisy and cumbersome. Humidification can be problematic.

3. High frequency IPPV
Conventional IPPV delivered at rates of 60 or more. It may occasionally be valuable but has little advantage over conventional forms of ventilation.

WEANING FROM ARTIFICIAL VENTILATION

As the patient's condition improves artificial ventilation can gradually be reduced until the patient is able to breathe on his/her own. The decision to start weaning is largely clinical, based on improving respiratory function and resolving underlying pathology (See Table 4.4). The need for further surgery, for example, may make weaning a futile exercise.

TABLE 4.4 Criteria for weaning

Haemodynamic	No arrhythmias	
	Minimal inotrope requirement	
	Optimal fluid balance	
Respiratory	FiO_2	<0.5
	$(A–a)DO_2$	<40–45 kPa
	Vital capacity	>10 ml/kg
	Tidal volume	>5 ml/kg
	Respiratory rate	<35
	Can generate negative inspiratory pressure	>20 cm H_2O
Metabolic	Normal acid base balance	pH<7.35
	Normal electrolytes	
	Normal CO_2 production	
	Normal oxygen demands	

There is no widely agreed policy on the best way to wean patients from ventilation. A typical approach is listed below.

● SIMV. Reduce the rate to allow the patient to take more breaths. Provide adequate pressure support and 5 cm H_2O of PEEP to reduce the work of breathing.
● When the patient is taking an adequate number of breaths, switch to CPAP, with pressure support.
● If the patient manages well gradually reduce the level of pressure support further. When the pressure support is down to 10 cm H_2O do not reduce it any further since the patient will have to work hard to overcome the resistance of the ventilator. Switch the patient to a separate flow generator CPAP system, so that they are on CPAP only.
● Finally reduce the CPAP so that the patient is just on a T-piece breathing humidified oxygen.
● Extubate at any stage when it is clear that the patient will cope.

Some patients, particularly postoperative elective surgical cases, will tolerate weaning well and can be rapidly extubated. Others, particularly those who have been ventilated for some time, or who have significant lung damage or muscle wasting, may take longer. They will often manage only a few hours or even minutes on CPAP and pressure support before getting tired, as indicated by sweating, increasing pulse rate and increasing respiratory rate (rapid shallow breaths). These patients then need a few hours' rest on the ventilator before starting to wean again. There is a growing role for non-invasive ventilation for weaning patients with COAD or neuromuscular disease.

PNEUMONIA

Pneumonia is defined as infection occurring in terminal respiratory airways. The pattern of illness and pathogens responsible depend on whether the infection was acquired in the community or in hospital, and on the patient's immune status. Community acquired pneumonias can be divided into those of 'typical' and 'atypical' presentation.

TYPICAL PNEUMONIA

Features of a 'typical' pneumonia include the following:

● Sudden onset of fever with rigors.
● Cough productive of mucopurulent sputum.
● Shortness of breath.
● Pleuritic chest pain.

Chest X-rays show the appearances of consolidation which may affect a single lobe, a whole lung or both lungs. The diagnosis is confirmed by raised WCC (predominantly neutrophils), and by results of sputum and blood culture. The causative organisms are commonly *Streptococcus pneumoniae* and *Haemophilus influenzae*. *Streptococcus pneumoniae* in particular may be associated with a generalized sepsis syndrome. *Staphylococcus* is less common.

ATYPICAL PNEUMONIA

Atypical pneumonias are so called because their mode of presentation is different from that seen in classic pneumonia. In particular the following presentations occur.

- Present over a few days compared to 24–36 hours of classic pneumonia.
- Non-respiratory symptoms dominate. Fever, malaise, myalgias and arthralgias common.
- Cough may only appear after a few days. Often non-productive. Sputum which is produced is clear and often negative on Gram stain and culture.
- Disparity between the clinical signs on chest examination and the CXR. Often minimal signs on examination of the chest, whilst CXR shows widespread patchy consolidation with interstitial and alveolar infiltrates.
- WCC may be normal or mildly elevated.

Causes of atypical pneumonia

Atypical penumonia
- Influenza A, B
- Parainfluenza
- Respiratory syncytial virus
- Pneumococcus
- *Legionella*
- Mycoplasma
- *Chlamydia*
- *Coxiella*
- *Leptospira*
- Tuberculosis

Whilst the list of causes is not exhaustive it gives an indication of the range of pathogens which may be responsible. The difficulty is often in making the diagnosis. You should seek advice from the microbiologist regarding investigations and treatment. The features of some atypical pneumonias are described below.

Mycoplasma pneumonia

Mycoplasma pneumonia is a community acquired infection which tends to affect young adults. It may progress to a multisystem disease with the following features:

- haemolytic anaemia, thrombocytopenia
- pericarditis, myocarditis, rarely endocarditis
- meningitis, encephalitis, peripheral and central nerve palsies
- vomiting and diarrhoea, hepatitis
- rashes myalgias and arthralgias.

The diagnosis is confirmed by rising antibody titre. Cold agglutinins occur in up to 50% of patients although this is non-specific and can occur in other atypical pneumonias notably *Legionella*.

Legionella pneumonia

Legionella may occur in outbreaks associated with infected showers and water cooling systems, but also occurs sporadically, particularly among older patients. Typical features are:

- prodromal flu-like illness
- dry cough
- fever up to 40°C associated with rigors
- nausea, vomiting diarrhoea and abdominal pain
- mental confusion
- haematuria and renal failure may develop
- multilobar shadowing and small pleural effusions on CXR.

The diagnosis is confirmed by rising antibody titre. *Legionella* may be identified by immunoflouresence on sputum, bronchial washings and urine.

MANAGEMENT OF PNEUMONIA

Investigations are summarized in Table 4.5 below. Not all patients require the full spectrum of special investigations.

TABLE 4.5 Investigations for pneumonia	
Sample	**Investigation**
Sputum (tracheal aspirate)	MC & S
B.A.L.*	MC & S (including AAFB)
	Legionella immunofluorescent antibody
	Viruses
	Fungi
	Pneumocystis carini
Nasopharyngeal aspirate	Viruses
Blood	Blood cultures (bacterial viral and fungal)
	Serology
	Viral titres
	Complement fixation (*Mycoplasma, Leptospirosis, Brucellosis*)
*See Practical procedures, bronchial alveolar lavage, p 259.	

The treatment of any pneumonia is twofold.

● Supportive therapy including humidified oxygen and ventilation as necessary. Regular physiotherapy and tracheal suction to aid clearance of secretions.
● Antibiotic therapy. This will depend upon the clinical picture and the nature of the infecting organism. Wherever possible microbiological specimens should be obtained prior to the commencement of antibiotics (see Table 4.6).

TABLE 4.6 Antibiotic therapy in community acquired pneumonia

Likely pathogen	Antibiotic
Streptoccocus pneumoniae *Haemophilus influenzae* (Atypical not excluded)	Cefuroxime & erythromycin
Staphylococcus	Flucloxacillin
Mycoplasma pneumoniae	Erythromycin 500 mg 6 hourly*
Legionella	Erythromycin 500 mg 6 hourly plus Rifampicin 1.2 g daily in divided doses (BD)*

*In atypical pneumonia antibiotic therapy should be continued for a minimum of 14 days.

NOSOCOMIAL PNEUMONIA

Up to 20% of all mechanically ventilated patients develop nosocomial or hospital acquired pneumonia although the incidence is higher in the immunocompromised patient. Gram-negative organisms and *Staphylococcus aureus* are particularly common.

A number of factors may increase the risk of nosocomial pneumonia in critically ill patients, by impairing host defence mechanisms and increasing colonization of the upper airway. These are summarized in Table 4.7.

TABLE 4.7 Factors predisposing to nosocomial pneumonia

Critical illness	Impaired host defences and immune systems
Sedation	Immune suppression Impaired mucus transport and cough mechanisms
Endotracheal & tracheostomy tubes	Bypass normal host defence mechanisms Increased colonization of upper airways Laryngeal incompetence increases the risk of aspiration
Nasogastric tubes	Increased colonization of upper airway with gut flora, particularly in the presence of reduced gastric acidity.
Effect of broad-spectrum antibiotics	Destroy normal commensal respiratory tract flora allowing pathogenic microorganisms to become established

Since little can be done to improve host defence mechanisms in the critically ill, ventilated patient, the best approach to reducing the incidence of nosocomial infection is to prevent contamination of the airway with pathogenic bacteria, in particular, by reducing the incidence of colonization of the upper airway. Ensure adequate hygiene procedures and aseptic technique at all times, e.g. always wear sterile gloves when suctioning the airway.

Maintenance of gastric acidity

The maintenance of a normal gastric pH is a major barrier to the colonization of the upper airway with gut flora, occurring via nasogastric tubes or the reflux of gastric contents. The use of H_2 blockers, such as ranitidine to reduce gastric acidity and prevent stress ulceration is therefore undesirable. Use sucralfate as an alternative. (See Stress ulcer prophylaxis p. 39.)

Selective decontamination digestive tract (SDD)

SDD is a method to reduce colonization of the upper airways by using oral, non-absorbable antibiotics, in an attempt to reduce the bacterial load in the GI tract. The evidence that this is effective at reducing nosocomial infection is limited, and at the current time SDD is not in widespread use.

Management of nosocomial infection

The management of nosocomial pneumonia is the same as for the management of any pneumonia (see above). Ideally antibiotics should be used only for microbiologically proven infection. If, however, the patient's condition dictates blind antibiotic therapy ensure microbiological specimens are obtained before commencing treatment. Antibiotic therapy needs to be guided by the likely source of the pathogens and by the local pattern of microbial antibiotic resistance. Table 4.8 is a guide.

TABLE 4.8 Empirical antibiotic therapy

Likely pathogens	Antibiotic
Strep pneumoniae Haemophilus influenzae Enterobacteria	Cefuroxime (if previously treated ciprofloxacin or ceftazidime)
Staphylococcus	Add flucloxacillin
Anaerobes	Add metronidazole

PNEUMONIA IN IMMUNOCOMPROMISED PATIENTS

(See also Haematology, the immunocompromised patient, p. 161.)
Patients who are immunocompromised for any reason, may present with pneumonia. In addition to the typical and atypical conditions already described a number of other opportunistic pathogens typically infect these patients.

Opportunistic infections

- *Pneumocystis carinii*
- Cytomegalovirus (CMV)
- Herpes virus (simplex & zoster)
- *Candida*
- *Aspergillus*

Pneumocystis carinii pneumonia (PCP)

Typical features are:

- fever
- dry cough
- breathlessness and severe hypoxaemia
- bilateral diffuse alveolar and interstitial shadowing.

80% of PCP can be detected by bronchial alveolar lavage (BAL). Occasionally transbronchial biopsy may be necessary. Treatment is high dose co-trimoxazole. Initiation of high-dose co-trimoxazole therapy should be covered by steroids to prevent acute lung inflammation.

- co-trimoxazole: 120 mg/kg daily in divided doses
- 0.5 g methylprednisolone daily for 3 days.

Cytomegalovirus (CMV)

CMV pneumonitis in immunocompromised patients is generally part of a disseminated infection in which there is also encephalitis, retinitis and involvement of the gastrointestinal tract. Cytology (BAL washings or biopsy) may show characteristic inclusion bodies. Diagnosis may be made by polymerase chain reaction (PCR), fluorescent antibody tests and tissue culture.

- intravenous ganciclovir 5 mg/kg 12 hourly

Fungal pneumonia

Colonization of the pharynx, gastrointestinal tract, perineum, wounds and skin folds is common and rarely requires treatment. Significant fungal infections may occur after prolonged treatment with antibiotics and particularly in immunocompromised patients. Infection is suggested by significant growth in sputum, tracheal aspirates, bronchial alveolar lavage fluids and blood cultures. In addition there may be rising serum antibody titres to candida or the presence of *Aspergillus* antigens. Fungal infection particularly fungal septicaemia is associated with a high mortality.

- amphoterecin B. 250 µg/kg daily initially increased to 1.2 mg/kg daily

ASPIRATION PNEUMONITIS

Patients with impaired conscious levels, impaired cough and gag reflexes, and susceptibility to regurgitation or vomiting are at risk of aspiration of gastric contents into the airway.

Aspiration may present with acute airway obstruction if the aspirated matter is solid. More commonly it presents as gradual onset of respiratory distress and respiratory failure either due to bacterial infection of the lungs or due to the inflammatory effects of acid aspiration. Up to a third of patients with known aspiration will develop ARDS (see ARDS, p. 98).

Therefore, if a patient is known to have aspirated gastric contents, for example, during an anaesthetic, manage them as follows.

- Suction the trachea to remove debris.
- Monitor clinical condition and oxygen saturation. Give humidified oxygen as required.
- Avoid antibiotics unless there is evidence of infection. If necessary antibiotic therapy should cover the normal respiratory pathogens plus Gram negatives and anaerobes. A combination of broad-spectrum cephalosporin and metronidazole is appropriate initially. Further treatment should be guided by the results of microbiological investigation.
- There is no role for prophylactic corticosteroids.
- Treat bronchospasm appropriately. (See asthma below.)
- If the patient's condition deteriorates ventilatory support may be necessary. If possible suction the trachea before any form of positive pressure ventilation is applied.

ASTHMA

Asthma occurs principally in young people. The incidence of this life threatening condition is increasing. Asthma involves increased airway reactivity, often triggered by an environmental stimulus, or following infection. An inflammatory process results in narrowing of small airways, mucus plugging, expiratory wheeze and air trapping. Asthma is a medical emergency. It may be rapidly progressive and clinical signs may be misleading. Severe cases may prove refractory even with maximal therapy and ventilation – do not underestimate its potential severity.

Clinical signs – severe asthma

- Cannot talk
- Tachypnoea, bradypnoea
- Tachycardia
- Pulsus paradox
- Recession
- Accessory muscle breathing
- 'Silent' chest

Management

- Monitor oxygen saturation continually. Give uncontrolled humidified oxygen. Asthmatics die from rapidly progressing unnoticed hypoxia.

- Commmence IV fluid, e.g. dex 4% saline 0.18%.
- Give nebulized β agonists (salbutamol 2.5–5 mg neb) and anticholinergics (ipratropium bromide 0.5 mg neb). Ensure nebulizers are given in oxygen not air.
- Give IV corticosteroids to suppress the inflammatory response. Hydrocortisone 200 mg bolus then 100 mg 6 hourly.
- There is no role for antibiotics unless there is clear evidence of a precipitating bacterial infection.
- If no improvement give IV β agonist, aminophylline 5 mg/kg loading dose IV over 10 minutes (unless already on theophyllines), followed by aminophylline infusion 0.5 mg/kg/min. Alternatively salbutamol 4 mg IV. Loading dose over 10 minutes followed by salbutamol infusion 5 μg min.
- If no improvement consider the need for mechanical ventilation.

Asthma: indications for ventilation
Exhaustion
Pa_{O_2} <6.5 kPa
Pa_{CO_2} >6.5 kPa
pH <7.3
Cardiorespiratory arrest

- When ventilating asthmatics always ensure adequate analgesia and sedation. The presence of an endotracheal tube in the larynx of an inadequately sedated asthmatic is a potent source of irritation and continued bronchoconstriction.

 Warning! The usual response to asthma is hyperventilation and a low Pa_{CO_2}. If Pa_{CO_2} starts to rise this is a grave sign indicating exhaustion of the patient and the imminent need for ventilation.

Ventilation in asthma

Positive pressure ventilation (IPPV) of asthmatics can be hazardous. Severe bronchoconstriction may result in prolonged expiratory time with resultant air trapping and hyperinflation. This in turn may produce both an inability to ventilate the patient adequately using conventional ventilator settings and the possibility of barotrauma due to high airway pressures, with the development of pneumothorax.

Therefore, in order to minimize these problems the ventilator settings may be adjusted to try and allow adequate time for expiration. The best combination of ventilation settings in any individual patient will be best determined by trial.

In general set a slow rate and prolonged expiratory time (I:E, 1:3–4) to allow adequate time for full expiration. The short inspiratory time may result in higher peak airway pressure. This is partially offset by the slower rate. In severe cases it may be necessary to accept raised Pa_{CO_2} rather than increase inspiratory pressures.

The role of PEEP in asthma is controversial. In theory adding PEEP increases FRC and actually worsens air trapping in patients who are hyperinflated. Alternatively high levels of PEEP have been used to splint open airways and improve ventilation. In practice try adding PEEP cautiously and see what the response is.

If hyperinflation becomes a problem it may be necessary to disconnect the patient from the ventilator momentarily and manually compress the chest wall to expel trapped air and improve respiratory mechanics. In reality the problem is rare.

 Warning! Sudden deterioration in a ventilated asthmatic should be assumed to be due to pneumothorax until proven otherwise.

CHRONIC OBSTRUCTIVE AIRWAYS DISEASE (COAD)

COAD disease is a broad term applied to patients with chronic bronchitis and emphysema. These conditions frequently coexist, and ultimately result in respiratory failure, episodes of which may be precipitated by intercurrent viral or bacterial respiratory infection.

Acute exacerbation of COAD

Patients with so-called acute exacerbations of COAD are generally managed on the medical ward with a combination of antibiotics, bronchodilators, controlled oxygen therapy (usually 24–35% oxygen by a fixed performance, Venturi system) and/or non-invasive ventilation. If despite this, their condition continues to deteriorate then you may be asked to assess them for ventilation. You should consider the following:

● These patients often tolerate markedly deranged blood gases very well. Therefore, it is the clinical condition of the patient that determines the need for ventilatory support. Assess the patient clinically. If they are able to talk, and are not distressed, they are unlikely to need immediate ventilation regardless of the blood gas picture.
● Hypoxia is usually the main problem. Consider increasing the inspired oxygen concentration.
● In some patients with COAD and type 2 respiratory failure, chronic hypercapnia results in loss of the normal ventilatory responsiveness to CO_2. In these patients hypoxia is the main stimulus to respiration. Giving high concentrations of inspired oxygen can result in the loss of the stimulus to

respiration and respiratory arrest. This situation is however, rare. Look at the bicarbonate on the blood gas. If this is normal, or only slightly raised (< 30 mmol/l) then chronic CO_2 retention does not exist and, therefore, the patient is not dependant on hypoxic drive. Increase the inspired oxygen concentration as necessary and repeat the blood gases after half an hour. In cases where hypoxic drive is genuinely the limiting factor then ventilation may be precipitated earlier.

● Avoid respiratory stimulants such as doxapram. These generally add little and can result in patients becoming exhausted and requiring ventilation. Only use as an interim measure to allow transport to an intensive care bed or when a decision has been made not to ventilate a patient (see below).

● If the patient remains severely hypoxic, becomes increasingly hypercapnic or clinically exhausted, urgent ventilation is likely to be necessary.

● Most patients with acute exacerbations of COAD who require a short period of ventilation do well and leave hospital. Patients in end stage respiratory failure, however, particularly those that have been ventilated before and who have been difficult to wean from ventilators, may not be suitable for further admission to intensive care. This decision should be taken by a senior doctor. If in doubt ask advice.

Warning! If the patient is in extremis there may not be time for a full assessment. In this case you should institute appropriate resuscitative measures including ventilation without delay.

Intensive care management

These patients are typically very distressed and have a high level of sympathetic catecholamine activity. Anaesthetic drugs used to intubate may abolish this and unmask relative hypovolaemia with subsequent cardiovascular collapse. Therefore:

● Where possible transfer the patient directly to the ICU for intubation and ventilation rather than attempting this on the ward.

● If the patient's condition allows, site arterial line and institute invasive pressure monitoring before induction. (CVP or pulmonary artery catheter can be placed later as necessary.)

● Consider giving 500 ml of fluid (e.g. Gelofusin) and have adrenaline available for resuscitation.

● After securing the airway institute IPPV. SIMV mode is usually adequate. Avoid hyperventilation. Rapid lowering of the $PaCO_2$ may further reduce sympathetic drive and lower the blood pressure.

● Continue antibiotic therapy according to local protocol. (See Pneumonia, p. 88 and Empirical antibiotic therapy, 204.)

● Nebulized bronchodilators. Salbutamol 2.5 mg and ipratropium bromide 500 µg.

● Consider intravenous bronchodilator therapy. Aminophylline 5 mg/kg loading dose (if not on long-term theophylline and not already loaded), followed by infusion aminophylline 0.5 mg/kg/h. Check levels.

● Corticosteroids. Hydrocortisone 200 mg initially then 100 mg 6 hourly.

Many of these patients require just a short period of ventilation and wean easily from the ventilator. Some, however, particularly those with type 2 respiratory failure may be more difficult to wean. In this group, early tracheostomy may be considered to improve patient comfort, and facilitate tracheal toilet, whilst allowing a reduction in sedative drugs.

● If there is difficulty weaning from ventilation: you may have to accept a raised $Pa\text{CO}_2$/reduced $Pa\text{O}_2$

ADULT RESPIRATORY DISTRESS SYNDROME (ARDS)

ARDS is a syndrome of acute respiratory failure characterized by an appropriate history of insult, marked respiratory distress with severe hypoxaemia, reduced pulmonary compliance and diffuse pulmonary infiltrates (non-cardiogenic pulmonary oedema) on CXR.

Pathophysiology

A large number of conditions are associated with the onset of ARDS (see Table 4.9). The exact mechanisms by which these conditions lead to lung injury are not fully understood. There is, however, an increased permeability of the alveolar capillaries which leak proteinacious fluid into the alveoli. This results in so-called 'non-cardiogenic pulmonary oedema.' This proteinaceous material precipitates, forming hyaline membranes and there is proliferation of inflammatory cells. Gradually the acute inflammatory process subsides and healing may occur. This may result in widespread interstitial lung fibrosis.

TABLE 4.9 Conditions associated with ARDS

Physical	Infective	Immune
Trauma	Septicaemia	Any severe illness
Head injury	Pneumonia	Blood transfusion
Blast injury		Cardiopulmonary
Acid aspiration		Bypass
Fat embolism		Anaphylaxis
Smoke inhalation		
Drugs		

Diagnosis

The clinical signs are those of increasing respiratory distress, with associated tachycardia, tachynpoea, and onset of cyanosis. Blood gases indicate severe hypoxaemia. The CXR shows acute bilateral interstitial and alveolar shadowing. The non-cardiogenic nature of the alveolar oedema can be confirmed by pulmonary artery catheterization. (PAOP < 18 mmHg, CI > 2L/min/m^3.) Infective processes may be excluded by BAL.

Management

- Treat the underlying cause.
- Invasive cardiovascular monitoring (arterial line/pulmonary artery catheter) and use of inotropes is appropriate in order to optimize cardiac output and oxygen delivery.
- Artificial ventilation is generally necessary. Reduced pulmonary compliance results in high inflation pressures, which are associated with increased barotrauma. Pressure control ventilation, with reversed I:E ratio (I:E, 2:1) may be used to limit peak airway pressure. Adequate sedation and paralysis may be helpful. PEEP is generally necessary to maintain oxygenation. High levels may be associated with reduced venous return and cardiac output and a worsening of oxygen delivery.
- The FiO_2 should be kept to the minimum necessary to maintain oxygenation, in order to reduce lung damage associated with oxygen free radicals. Moderate levels of hypercarbia may be tolerated (permissive hypercapnia) if excessive ventilatory pressures would otherwise be required.
- Nitric oxide is a naturally occurring substance produced from the endothelium of blood vessels which causes vasodilatation. If added to the inspiratory gases in concentrations of 5–20 vpm it results in pulmonary vasodilatation in those areas of the lung which are well ventilated. Blood is diverted away from poorly ventilated areas, the shunt fraction is reduced and there is an improvement in oxygenation. At the same time pulmonary hypertension and the risk of right heart failure is reduced. Nitric oxide has a short half-life when inhaled and is generally safe for the patient. It is, however, a toxic gas and should only be used according to the protocols established in your unit.
- Diuretics may be used to reduce the transpulmonary capillary pressure in an attempt to reduce the development of pulmonary oedema.
- Turning the patient prone may improve V/Q mismatch and blood gases. The benefit generally tends to be temporary (24–48 hours).
- Enteral feeding should commence as soon as possible.

INTERPRETING CHEST X-RAYS IN ICU

The combination of intubation or tracheostomy, and IPPV makes interpretation of classic respiratory signs in the noisy environment of the ICU very difficult. The CXR, therefore, assumes additional importance when evaluating the patient's condition.

You must be able to recognize the typical abnormal appearances seen in intensive care, particularly those which relate to complications of procedures. It is best, therefore, to have a standard system for evaluating the CXR.

● Check name, date and orientation of film. (Normal CXR orientation is P–A. That is the X-rays are passed through the patient from behind towards the film which is in front. Films taken in intensive care are generally A–P. (This alters the magnification of structures.)
● Check penetration and rotation of film.
● Check mediastinal structures, including cardiac shadow, lung hilum and pulmonary vessels. Check the position of tracheal tubes, central venous and pulmonary artery catheters, and also the position of any nasogastric tube.
● Check lung fields. Note position of diaphragms.
● Check bones and soft tissues.

A number of CXR patterns are common in intensive care.

1. Consolidation (→ Fig. 4.3)

● Opacification of a lobe or segment (may be patchy).
● No loss of lung volume.
● Mediastinal and diaphragmatic borders partially preserved.

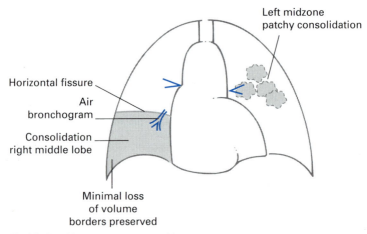

Fig. 4.3 Chest X-ray interpretation: consolidation.

2. Collapse of lobe (→ Fig. 4.4)

● Loss of volume on side of collapse.
● Compensatory hyperinflation of remaning lobes.
● Shift of mediastinal structures towards side of collapse.

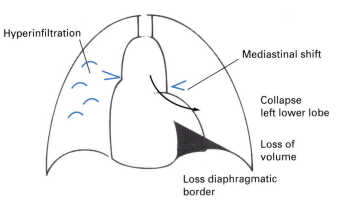

Fig. 4.4 Chest X-ray interpretation: collapse of lobe.

3. Collapse of a lung (→ Fig. 4.5)

- Loss of volume of collapsed side.
- Trachea and hilar structures pulled across.
- Diaphrgam obscured.
- Opposite lung hyperinflated.

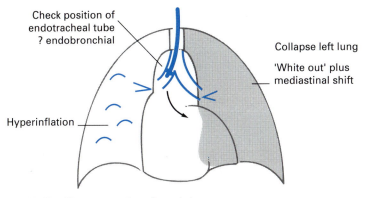

Fig. 4.5 Chest X-ray interpretation: collapse of a lung.

4. Pleural effusion/haemothorax (→ Fig. 4.6)

- In intensive care patients' CXRs are generally taken with the patient supine. Therefore the classic appearance of pleural effusions obscuring the costodiaphragmatic recess may be missed.
- Small effusions may produce general haze to whole lung field.
- Large effusions may produce shift of mediastinal structures to the other side.

Upright film   **Supine film**

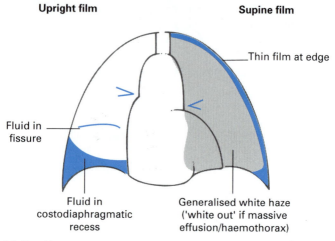

Thin film at edge

Fluid in fissure

Fluid in costodiaphragmatic recess

Generalised white haze ('white out' if massive effusion/haemothorax)

Fig. 4.6 Chest X-ray interpretation: pleural effusion/haemothorax.

5. Pulmonary oedema (→ Fig. 4.7)

● Typical features of pulmonary oedema may be altered by the effects of mechanical ventilation.
● Perihilar shadowing.
● Interstitial shadowing
● Marked airspace shadowing particularly in the lower zones.
● Fluid in the fissures and small pleural effusions.

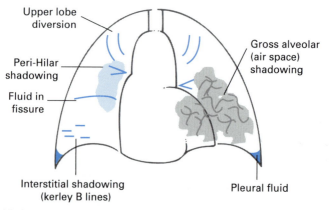

Upper lobe diversion

Gross alveolar (air space) shadowing

Peri-Hilar shadowing

Fluid in fissure

Interstitial shadowing (kerley B lines)

Pleural fluid

Fig. 4.7 Chest X-ray interpretation: pulmonary oedema.

6. Adult respiratory distress syndrome (→ Fig. 4.8)

The CXR features of ARDs are not specific. The common response to lung injury is leaking of capillaries, accumulation of alveolar fluid and subsequent development of areas of collapse and consolidation. The features are, therefore, a combination of those described above.

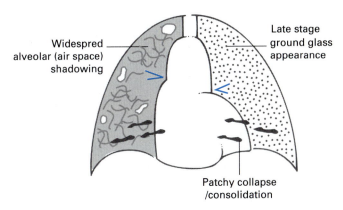

Fig. 4.8 Chest X-ray interpretation: adult respiratory distress syndrome.

7. Position of lines and tubes (→ Fig. 4.9)

All central lines, pulmonary artery catheters and tubes visible by CXR should be checked for correct placement and for the presence of any complications. This includes the following:

● Endotracheal tube, not endobronchial.
● Central venous lines. Intravascular and the tip positioned in the superior vena cava, above the pericardial reflections.
● Pulmonary artery catheter. Tip lying in the pulmonary artery, preferably on the right side and not too distal.
● Nasogastric tube in the stomach.

8. Pneumothorax (→ Fig. 4.10)

Pneumothorax should be suspected in any patient who deteriorates whilst on a ventilator, particularly if there is associated trauma, or recent central line insertion.

● Typical pattern is of visible lung edge and translucent free air in the pleural space.
● In the supine patient air may lie anteriorly over the medisatinal structures and the lung edge appear normal. Suspect this if there is anterior translucency (blackness). A lateral CXR may help.

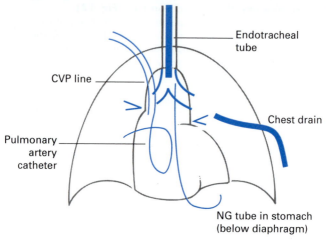

Endotracheal tube

CVP line

Pulmonary artery catheter

Chest drain

NG tube in stomach (below diaphragm)

Fig. 4.9 Chest X-ray interpretation: position of lines and tubes.

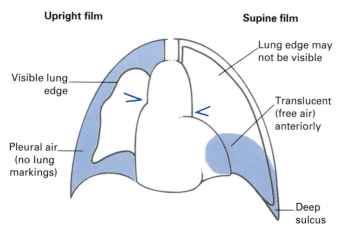

Upright film

Supine film

Visible lung edge

Pleural air (no lung markings)

Lung edge may not be visible

Translucent (free air) anteriorly

Deep sulcus

Fig. 4.10 Chest X-ray interpretation: pneumothorax.

9. Trauma (→ Fig. 4.11)

● Check for fractured ribs. If present think about the injury to the underlying structures. For fractures of ribs 1–3 consider injury to subclavian vessels (haemothorax). For fractures of ribs 9–12 consider injury to the liver or spleen.
● For all rib fractures consider the underlying lung injury and evidence of lung contusion.
● Evidence of sternal fractures. Consider myocardial injury.
● Evidence of mediastinal injury, particularly widened mediastinum which suggests major vascular injury and requires expert assessment and intervention.

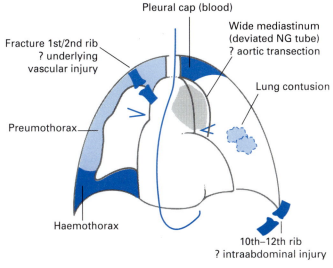

Fig. 4.11 Chest X-ray interpretation: trauma.

CHAPTER 5

GASTROINTESTINAL SYSTEM

GASTROINTESTINAL SYSTEM

There is increasing interest in the role of the gut in critical illness. Aside from absorption of nutrients the gut is important as follows:

● As a large third space for fluid losses both in gut disease and conditions with generalized capillary leak.
● As a potential source for bacteria/endotoxins which may colonize the respiratory tract and other sites or translocate into the portal and systemic circulation.
● Site for AV shunting (low SVR) in sepsis states. (See Sepsis: pathophysiology, p. 200.)

GASTROINTESTINAL TRACT FAILURE

The maintenance of gastrointestinal integrity and function is of major importance. Aggressive early resuscitation with fluids and use of dopexamine or dopamine may help to preserve splanchnic perfusion, the adequacy of which can be monitored using gastric tonometry. Early enteral nutrition may also help to preserve mucosal integrity. (See Gastric tonometry, p. 264 and Enteral feeding p. 36.)

Failure of the gastrointestinal tract during critical illness may present in a number of ways.

Clinical features of GI tract failure

● Failure to absorb feed
● Delayed gastric emptying
● Stress ulceration
● Ileus, pseudo-obstruction
● Diarrhoea.
● Acalculous cholecystitis
● Liver dysfunction
● SIRS

Stress ulceration

This may occur in either the duodenum or stomach resulting in bleeding or actual perforation of the ulcer. It is thought to be primarily due to inadequacy of mucosal blood flow. General resuscitation measures including adequate fluid loading and use of dopexamine or dopamine to increase splanchnic perfusion are more important than prophylactic measures.

Perforation needs to be considered in patients with abdominal signs who deteriorate. Diagnosis is generally made by seeing free air on plain abdominal film. Seek surgical opinion. (See Stress ulcer prophylaxis, p. 39 and GI bleeding, p. 110.)

Persistent ileus and pseudo-obstruction

Failure of gut motility is common in the critically ill. This is most commonly manifest as a simple ileus with failure to absorb feed and large nasogastric losses. This will usually improve spontaneously as the patient's condition improves. Prokinetic agents such as cisapride may promote the recovery of motility.

Occasionally ileus will progress to marked intraabdominal distention, with obvious signs of gut obstruction despite no obviously apparent mechanical cause. This is called pseudoobstruction.

The diagnosis is made by plain abdominal X-ray, which shows widely dilated loops of bowel. If the colon is distended to greater than 10–12 cm in cross-section, there is a risk of colonic rupture. The use of prokinetic agents in this setting may be hazardous and mechanical decompression is usually necessary to prevent colonic rupture. This may be achieved by flexible sigmoidoscopy, or may require surgical intervention. Seek surgical opinion.

Ischaemic bowel

This should be considered as a possible cause of deterioration particularly in the elderly patient with preexisting vascular disease or vasculitis. There are no specific clinical signs or special investigations although worsening sepsis, oliguria, persistent acidosis, a raised amylase and occasionally bloody diarrhoea are all features. The diagnosis may be suggested by CT scans showing gas in the gut wall. The diagnosis is usually made at laparotomy. Seek surgical opinion.

Acalculous cholecystitis

Cholestasis is common in the critically ill particularly in the absence of enteral feed. This may result in ascending cholangitis which sometimes requires antibiotic treatment.

Occasionally, critically ill patients may develope an acute, necrotizing inflammation of the gallbladder, or acalculous cholecystitis. The aetiology of this is multifactorial but includes bile stasis, and splanchnic hypoperfusion. It should be considered in any patient with progressive jaundice, abdominal signs and evidence of sepsis. Abdominal ultrasound will often demonstrate an enlarged, oedematous gallbladder. Management options include CT guided drainage and acute cholecystectomy. Seek surgical opinion.

Liver dysfunction during critical illness

Liver dysfunction (as oppposed to liver failure) is common during critical illness, particularly in association with severe shock states in which there is relative splanchnic and liver hypoperfusion. It is characterized by progressive rise in bilirubin, abnormalities of liver enzyme, coagulopathy with raised PT time and delayed drug metabolism. The management is essentially supportive. The liver function should improve as the patient's general condition improves.

Intraabdominal collections of pus

Subphrenic, pelvic and other intraabdominal collections are an ever-present threat in critically ill patients, particularly following any intraabdominal surgery. The clinical signs and symptoms may be vague. Persistent ileus, with failure to absorb feeds and 'grumbling' sepsis should raise suspicions. Assessment is by clinical examination followed by ultrasound or CT imaging. Management depends on the clinical condition of the patient but is radiologically guided, or open surgical drainage.

GASTROINTESTINAL BLEEDING

The term generally refers to massive bleeding from the upper GI tract. Lower GI bleeds occur less commonly; melaena or massive rectal bleeding may be of upper GI origin.

Causes of upper GI haemorrhage
Duodenal ulceration
Gastric erosion & ulceration
Oesophageal varices
Portal gastropathy
Aortoenteric fistulae
AV malformations
Other small bowel lesions

Clinical features

History may be suggestive of the underlying diagnosis – predisposing factors include previous peptic ulceration, non-steroidal anti-inflammatory drugs (NSAIDs), corticosteroids, anticoagulants, liver disease, portal hypertension and critical illness. Brisk GI bleeding is complicated by hypovolaemic shock and oliguria. Patients with liver disease develop worsening encephalopathy. Myocardial ischaemia may result and aspiration pneumonia may develop particularly where conscious level is obtunded.

Investigations

Full blood count and cross-match are followed by regular monitoring of haemodynamic status, urine output, haemoglobin, clotting screen and electrolytes. The site of the bleeding point is identified by endoscopy or arteriography.

Management

● Good vascular access is obtained and resuscitation of hypovolaemia commenced. CVP monitoring should be used to guide resuscitation. In massive bleeds full haemodynamic monitoring including arterial line and pulmonary artery catheterization is valuable. Goal-directed therapy may help to avoid multiorgan failure.

- Coagulopathy should be assessed and corrected.
- Analgesics and anxiolytics are used judiciously in conscious patients. Massive bleeds, however, frequently necessitate intubation and ventilation.
- Endoscopy allows injection of bleeding ulcers and banding or sclerotherapy of varices. The coadministration of a proton-pump inhibitor (e.g. omeprazole 40 mg once or twice daily) is frequently all that is required to prevent recurrence. However, persistent uncontrollable GI bleeding may necessitate surgery.
- Persistent variceal bleeding carries a high mortality (up to 50% from a first presentation). Measures to reduce portal hypertension include the administration of vasopressin (up to 20 units by s.c. injection or slow IV infusion: beware vasopressor effects) and octreotide.
- Linton or Sengstaken–Blakemore tubes possess a balloon to compress varices in the gastric fundus. If such measures are ineffective, specialist surgical techniques may be required. These include splenorenal shunting, mesocaval shunting, oesophageal transection and liver transplantation. Such drastic interventions carry a high mortality. (See Practical procedures: Sengstaken–Blakemore tube, p. 265.)

FULMINANT HEPATIC FAILURE

Liver failure is defined as hyperacute where the onset of encephalopathy occurs within 7 days of the onset of jaundice, acute where the interval is 7–28 days and subacute where it is between 28 days and 6 months. Longer intervals represent chronic liver failure. The term fulminant liver failure refers to an earlier classification where encephalopathy occurs within 8 weeks of the onset of jaundice. It thus encompasses acute and hyperacute liver failure.

Aetiology

The commonest cause worldwide remains hepatitis B. In the UK this is second to paracetamol poisoning. Other common causes include hepatitis A, drug idiosyncrasy and non-A, non-B viral hepatitis. (Note: this does not equate to hepatitis C, which is not thought to be a cause of fulminant liver failure. Up to 20% of cases may however be hepatitis E.)

Pathophysiology

The final common pathway is hepatocellular failure with a reduction or loss of the synthetic, homeostatic and filter functions of the liver. This results in a failure of carbohydrate metabolism in association with a depletion of glycogen stores and consequent hypoglycaemia. Deranged amino-acid metabolism results in accumulation of ammonia and other intermediate compounds which account in part for the development of encephalopathy.

Protein synthesis is arrested, and this includes the synthesis of albumin and clotting factors. Coagulopathy is invariable. Prothrombin time (PT) is the most sensitive index of hepatocellular failure and recovery. The coagulopathy may be exacerbated by activated fibrinolysis.

The filter (reticuloendothelial) functions of the hepatic Kupffer cells are central to the prevention of translocation of gut-derived endotoxin to the systemic circulation. In acute liver failure, there is systemic endotoxaemia. Further, the massive necrosis of hepatocytes releases high levels of tumour necrosis factor (TNF), PAF and other proinflammatory cytokines. Triggering of the inflammatory cascade, the systemic inflammatory response syndrome (SIRS) and multisystem organ failure (MOF) thus ensue. The classic 'septic' haemodynamic picture is associated with this.

The combination of these effects gives rise to failure of the blood–brain barrier with cerebral oedema and altered consciousness.

Clinical features

The clinical features reflect the pathophysiology. Hypoglycaemia is common, and develops any time in the first few days of the condition. It gradually resolves as the liver failure improves. Acid base homoeostasis is altered and either alkalosis or acidosis may complicate this. A metabolic acidosis is the more sinister.

Concurrently with the development of the metabolic derangement, conscious level may become impaired. Encephalopathy is graded as in Table 5.1.

TABLE 5.1 Grade hepatic encephalopathy

0	Normal
1	Mild confusion. (may not be immediately evident)
2	Drowsiness, worsening confusion
3	Severe drowsiness, inappropriate words/phrases, grinding teeth.
4	Unrousable

The onset of encephalopathy is followed in some patients by cerebral oedema and raised intracranial pressure (ICP). The risk of raised ICP is greatest in hyperacute liver failure (in excess of 50% of cases), and much lower in acute failure. It is virtually unknown to complicate subacute failure. A baseline elevation in ICP up to 20–25 mmHg may be followed by surges, which are transient but severe (up to 80–90 mmHg). This stage may be followed by inexorably rising ICP and brain death.

The haemodynamics of SIRS develop as conscious level reaches grade III–IV. The characteristic hypotension is associated with a high cardiac index and low systemic vascular resistance. Vasodilatation and increased capillary permeability contribute to reduced circulating volume and may predispose to renal failure. Acute tubular necrosis may also occur as a result of SIRS or directly as a result of the precipitating insult, e.g. paracetamol-induced renal damage.

The coagulopathy seldom gives rise to de novo bleeding, even though very high PT values are seen (> 100 s). Generalized oozing around cannulation sites is common but is seldom of great significance. Thrombocytopenia may also occur, either due to DIC or hypersplenism. It is occasionally necessary to perform invasive procedures under platelet cover.

True 'infective' sepsis may follow intubation and the insertion of invasive monitoring. A rising leucocyte count, falling platelet count, a PT whose recovery becomes arrested or a worsening acidosis must all be regarded as suspicious.

Management

 Warning! Hepatic failure carries a high mortality. Treatment options include liver transplantation, so hepatic failure is best managed in specialist centres where experience is concentrated. Early referral and discussion with a specialist centre are mandatory.

The predictive factors for best outcome with medical treatment versus liver transplantation can be complex and are dependent on the course of the disease as well as the underlying diagnosis. Medical management frequently has a role even in those with grade IV encephalopathy. Metabolic status must be closely monitored.

- All infusions are made up in dextrose solutions (5–20%) and dextrose (5–50%) infused to maintain a normal blood sugar.
- Nitrogenous feeds are avoided (no TPN or nasogastric feed should be administered until metabolic resolution of acute liver failure).
- Sodium and potassium are maintained within the normal range; this may involve slow judicious use of potassium infusions 10–40 mmol/h.
- Metabolic acidosis is a useful prognostic indicator and is in any case best left untreated on theoretical grounds. The exception to this is where a severe acidosis is associated with haemodynamic instability. It is acceptable to correct the pH slowly to 7.2 if this improves the haemodynamic status. Tris-buffered solution or carbicarb are preferable to sodium bicarbonate as the risks of paradoxical intracellular acidosis and hypernatraemia are less.

 Warning! PT is the most sensitive index of the evolution of the disease process and is frequently the key prognostic indicator determining whether the optimal management is likely to be medical or liver transplantation. Even ICP bolt placement is performed in many transplant centres without fresh frozen plasma (FFP) supplementation. Therefore, do not treat coagulopathy except in the case of life threatening haemorrhage. You obscure the PT at your peril!

Worsening encephalopathy to grade III–IV and SIRS are both indications for mechanical ventilation. This protects the airway, reduces the work of breathing and protects against the risk of secondary hypoxic damage. ICP must be monitored in at-risk patients. Surges in ICP are prevented by appropriate sedation and paralysis and by neurologically aware nursing protocols. The patient is nursed at a 20° head-up tilt. Turning, physiotherapy and tracheal suctioning are avoided until the risk of ICP surges resolves (usually 5 days after the onset of grade IV encephalopathy).

● Ensure adequate sedation and paralysis, e.g infusions of propofol, alfentanil and atracurium.

● Fluid and haemodynamic management is guided by invasive monitoring with a pulmonary artery catheter. Maintain adequate filling to ensure optimal CO while avoiding the risk of interstitial oedema of the lung, brain and gut. A PAOP around 10–12 mmHg is generally reasonable.

● Adrenaline or noradrenaline are used to keep the mean arterial pressure above 70–80 mmHg and the CPP > 40–50 mmHg (see below).

● Dopamine or dopexamine at a renotropic dose may be used for splanchnic protection. Stress ulcer prophylaxis with an H_2 antagonist or sucralfate is important.

● Renal failure can present problems with fluid loading. Slow haemofiltration or haemodiafiltration are frequently necessary, but are often associated with transient haemodynamic instability and ICP surges.

● Antoxidant regimens are as yet unproved, though prolonged treatment with prostacyclin and N-acetylcysteine have both been shown to improve outcome in fulminant liver failure irrespective of aetiology, even when instituted relatively late in the disease process.

● The liver will not metabolize citrate used as an anticoagulant in blood products. This chelates calcium, and may drastically reduce ionized calcium levels. Calcium chloride 10 mmol may be given by slow bolus to raise the ionized calcium to above 0.8 mmol/l.

● The prevention of sepsis is a major problem. Prophylactic antibiotics should be discussed with a microbiologist. Selective digestive tract decontamination is currently thought to be of value.

● Primary surges in ICP (often followed by a reflex rise in arterial pressure) are treated acutely by hyperventilation. The response to hyperventilation is not maintained, so it should be discontinued as soon as a fall in ICP is seen. Mannitol 20% 100 ml is used to sustain the reduction in ICP and also where the baseline ICP remains above 25 mmHg. Even where the ICP remains very high a good neurological outcome is possible provided cerebral perfusion pressure (CPP) is maintained at or above 40–50 mmHg. The last resort measure in patients with a falling CPP is thiopentone coma.

Prognosis

Without transplantation, the prognosis is poorest in the subacute group and best in the hyperacute group. Within this group, the prognosis is poorer in those at the extremes of age, those with non-A non-B hepatitis and drug dyscrasia. The overall mortality in patients with grade IV encephalopathy is 70%.

With liver transplantation (i.e. in those patients at the highest risk of death with optimal medical management), the 1 year mortality is between 30–50%.

PANCREATITIS

Inflammation of the pancreas and autodigestion may be precipitated by a number of causes, the commonest of which are alcohol and biliary obstruction. Often, there is no obvious cause.

Causes of pancreatitis

Alcohol
Biliary obstruction (gallstones)
Viral infection (CMV, EBV, etc)
Surgical injury
Hypothermia
Corticosteroids
Oral contraceptives

Clinical features

A spectrum of severity exists from mild pain to severe shock. Epigastric pain radiating to the back and a history of risk factors (including previous episodes) suggest the diagnosis. Examination may reveal flank discolouration (Grey–Turner sign) and peritonism. SIRS, ARDS, coagulopathy and renal failure may develop. 'Soap formation' leads to hypocalcaemia and hypomagnesaemia, with hypotension and a tendency to tachyarrhythmias. Diabetes mellitus arising de novo may be permanent.

Investigations

Raised serum amylase (>1000 IU/l) is a diagnostic but often absent finding. Values in the range 100–1000 suggest alternative intraabdominal pathologies, including perforated viscus. Localized posterior perforations of duodenum or stomach may be difficult to distinguish. Chest and abdominal plain films should confirm the absence of free gas or pneumonia, and may show calcium deposition. In severe cases the typical radiographic features of ARDS may be present. Plain film and ultrasound may confirm the presence of gallstones or other underlying biliary lesion. Blood glucose and arterial gases should be closely monitored. As the condition progresses, serial CT scanning is valuable to diagnose and monitor cysts/pseudocysts.

Management

In milder forms, analgesia is the mainstay of treatment. Pethidine theoretically causes less spasm of the sphincter of Oddi than does morphine. Hyperglycaemia is managed by sliding scale insulin infusion. Traditionally, the GI tract is rested by insertion of a nasogastric tube and regular drainage/aspiration. Total parenteral nutrition is frequently introduced early in the condition. These views are currently undergoing reappraisal; some studies suggest that very early enteral feeding reduces mortality.

In some centres, octreotide (25 µg hourly by infusion) is used to reduce exocrine activity. Patients who develop SIRS/ARDS, require intubation, ventilation and haemodynamic optimization. These patients may benefit from antioxidant regimens. Acute renal failure may require renal replacement therapy. Particular attention should be paid to acid-base balance and electrolyte disorders. Calcium, phosphate and magnesium supplementation are often needed. Defficiencies of these electrolytes may be a recurring and severe problem.

Pancreatic cyst/pseudocyst formation requires expert surgical intervention. Treatment may be conservative, radiologically guided drainage or surgical excision. The latter may require repeated laparotomy for intraabdominal sepsis.

Prognosis

This depends on the severity of the disease and the occurrence of SIRS, ARDS and ARF. In general the prognosis is poorer in the elderly and in those with pre-existing diabetes mellitus.

RENAL SYSTEM

RENAL DYSFUNCTION

Renal dysfunction is common in the ICU and frequently occurs as part of a syndrome of multiple organ failure. It is usually manifest as oliguria progressing to anuria, but high-output renal failure, in which there are large volumes of poorly concentrated urine, may also be seen.

Patients in intensive care who develop acute renal failure (ARF) have a mortality rate around 50%. This high mortality rate probably reflects the seriousness of the underlying condition, rather than mortality specifically attributable to renal failure. Patients usually die with renal failure rather than from renal failure.

Aetiology

The causes of renal dysfunction can be divided into prerenal (inadequate perfusion), renal (intrinsic renal disease) and postrenal (obstruction). These are summarised in Table 6.1.

TABLE 6.1 Causes of renal failure

Prerenal	Renal	Postrenal
Dehydration	Renovascular disease	Mechanical obstruction kidney
Hypovolaemia	Autoimmune disease	Ureteric tumour, calculus
Hypotension	SIRS & sepsis	Bladder outlet obstruction
	Jaundice/haemaglobinuria	
	Crush injury (myoglobinuria)	
	Nephrotoxic drugs	

In intensive care patients, the causes of renal dysfunction are often multifactorial with prerenal and renal factors combined. Preexisting intrinsic renal impairment is compounded by the effects of critical illness including release of cytokines, hypoperfusion, altered tissue oxygen delivery/extraction, and altered cellular function. In addition many drugs used in intensive care are predictably nephrotoxic while others have been implicated in idiosyncratic nephrotoxic reactions.

Terminology

Prerenal failure. This refers to decreased glomerular filtration rate (GFR) due to reduced perfusion. There is no tubular damage. Immediately reversed after adequate resuscitation/reperfusion.

Acute tubular necrosis (ATN). Decreased GFR due to reduced perfusion resulting in ischaemic renal tubular damage. No immediate reversal on restoration of perfusion. Usually improves over time.

Acute cortical necrosis (ACN). Rare syndrome with total and irreversible loss of renal function from severe prolonged ischaemia of kidneys. It is most commonly seen complicating pregnancy-related ARF.

INVESTIGATION OF ACUTE RENAL DYSFUNCTION

In many cases, the causes of acute renal dysfunction in the ICU can be determined from knowledge of the clinical background of the patient and by simple history and examination. Most cases of ARF will prove to be prerenal or acute tubular necrosis. Up to 10% of cases, however, will have other significant underlying pathologies.

History and examination

● Is there any indication of pre-existing renal disease? Vascular disease, diabetes, multisystem disease/vasculitis, chronic anaemia or previously abnormal U&Es are all suggestive. (Look for small shrunken kidneys on ultrasound or CT.)
● Is there any evidence for prerenal impairment? Dehydration, hypovolaemia, or hypotension.
● Is there any evidence for new intrinsic renal impairment? Sepsis, nephrotoxic drugs.
● Is there any history or evidence of trauma or obstruction to the GU tract?

Investigations

● Serial U & Es. These should not be taken as individual values, but viewed as a trend. Used to monitor renal function and predict the need for renal replacement therapy.
● Urinary U & Es.
● Urine and plasma osmolarity.
● Urine microscopy – are there casts, red cells, crystals?

Normal urine osmolality depends on the hydration status of the patient and may vary from hypoosmolar (less than normal plasma osmlality 280 mosm/l) to highly concentrated hyperosmolar (> 1000 mosmol/l).

In prerenal failure, the kidney is functioning maximally to retain sodium and water in order to re-expand plasma volume. The urine sodium concentration is low and the urine is maximally concentrated, as indicated by high osmolality (600–900 mosmol/l), and a urine–to–plasma urea ratio greater than 10.

As ATN develops, the renal tubules are no longer able to function normally, and are unable to retain sodium or concentrate the urine. The urinary sodium rises, urinary osmolality falls and the urine–to–plasma urea ratio also falls. Eventually the urinary sodium and osmolality would approach that of plasma. Renal tubular debris or casts may be seen in the urine.

TABLE 6.2 Features of prerenal and renal failure

	Prerenal	Renal (ATN)
Urinary sodium*	< 10 mmol/l	> 30 mmol/l
Urinary osmolality*	High	Low
Urinary/plasma Urea ratio*	> 10:1	< 8:1
Urine microscopy	Normal	Tubular casts

*NB: if patients have received diuretics this chemistry is difficult to interpret.

● Vasculitic screen: renal disease may be associated with autoimmune conditions and vasculitidies. An autoimmune/vasculitic screen may be appropriate particularly in the presence of coexisting pulmonary disease. Investigations are listed in Table 6.3.

TABLE 6.3 Investigations for autoimmune disease in renal failure

Vasculitis	Antineutrophil cytoplasmic antibodies (ANCA)
Goodpasture's syndrome	Antiglomerular basement membrane antibodies
Systemic lupus erythematosis (SLE)	Antinuclear antibodies (ANA) Antidouble-stranded DNA antibodies
Rheumatoid disease	Rheumatoid factor

● Plain abdominal films may show calcification or stones and give an impression of kidney size. Intravenous pyelogram (IVP) is not usually performed in ARF.
● Renal ultrasound may demonstrate small shrunken kidneys in cases with chronic renal failure. Ultrasound is useful to show obstruction (e.g. distended ureters or renal pelvis).
● CT scan with contrast may be useful in trauma/obstruction.
● Renal biopsy and radioisotope perfusion scans may be useful in difficult cases.

COMMON PROBLEM: OLIGURIA

Oliguria is defined as a urine output of less than 0.5 ml/kg/hour for at least two consecutive hours. Most cases of oliguria do not progress to ARF if adequate steps are taken.

 Warning! Check that the urinary catheter is not blocked, particularly if the oliguria is intermittent. Flushing catheters is not always sufficient. A few cases of 'renal failure' may be cured by recatheterization.

● Review the biochemistry results. Is there evidence of deteriorating renal function over time? (i.e. increasing serum urea and creatinine.)
● Review the clinical status of the patient.
● Is there evidence of dehydration/hypovolaemia suggested by: poor tissue turgor (pinch skin on back of hand), dry mouth, cool pale limbs, low CVP or wedge pressure, large respiratory swing on arterial line?
● Are CO and BP adequate?
● Is there any obvious cause for renal failure, e.g. chronic renal insufficiency, nephrotoxic drugs, rhabdomyolysis?

Management

● Give volume according to clinical signs. Even if the patient is apparently normovolaemic it is generally worth giving a fluid challenge (e.g. 500 ml colloid). Response may not be immediate. If there is no response consider the need for a PA catheter to further assess volume status.
● Commence low dose dopamine 1–3 µg/kg/min or dopexamine 1 µg/kg/min. This may improve renal perfusion and GFR.
● Renal filtration is a pressure-dependent process. Elderly patients, and, in particular, those with vascular disease, may require a higher than expected mean blood pressure. Consider the use of inotropes to generate a BP approaching the normal or admission BP for that patient. Vasopressors may improve urine output if perfusion pressure increases appropriately.
● If the cause of the oliguria is not clear from clinical evaluation and there is no response to simple measures then consider investigations above.
● Consider stopping nephrotoxic drugs, exclude undrained sources of sepsis, necrotic muscle (rhabdomyolysis) and ischaemic gut.
● Give bumetanide 1–2 mg bolus IV, or frusemide 20–40 mgs bolus IV. (Bumetanide may be preferable to frusemide since it does not require to be filtered by the glomerulus to achieve its effect.) If there is a response, consider the use of an infusion to maintain urine output. Bumetanide 1–2 mg/h or frusemide 20–40 mg/h.
● If there is no response, give bumetanide 5 mg or frusemide 250 mg over 1 hour. If there is a response, follow this with an infusion as above.

Warning! Urine output generated by diuretics may aid fluid balance, but not be adequate for maintaining acceptable biochemistry. Pay careful attention to fluid balance, and monitor biochemistry.

● If there is still no response then ARF is established. Restrict fluid intake to the previous hour's urine output plus 30–50 ml to allow for insensible losses. Seek advice and renal support. (See below.)

PROBLEMS OF ACUTE RENAL FAILURE (ARF)

The problems associated with ARF are inability to excrete fluid, impaired acid–base regulation, hyperkalaemia and accumulation of waste products.

● Inability to excrete fluid may result in progressive fluid overload. This may be manifest as hypertension and widespread tissue oedema. Pulmonary oedema may result in impaired gas exchange.
● Impaired acid–base balance results in accumulation of hydrogen ions and metabolic acidosis.
● Impaired excretion of potassium leads to hyperkalaemia. This can develop rapidly and is a medical emergency. Other problems of electrolyte disturbance include abnormalities of sodium, phosphate and calcium balance.
● Accumulation of creatinine, urea, and other middle molecules may produce clouding of conscious level, metabolic encephalopathy, and myocardial depression. GI side-effects include gastric stasis and ileus. Accumulation of middle molecules may contribute to a coagulopathy due to effects on platelet function.

MANAGEMENT OF ACUTE RENAL FAILURE (ARF)

The management of a patient in renal failure requires a multidisciplinary approach. You should seek advice from your renal physicians or local renal unit.

Control of hyperkalaemia
The main concern in the acute phase is the development of ventricular dysrhythmias associated with hyperkalaemia. Potassium levels can rise quickly in the presence of severe sepsis and hypercatabolism. Patients with chronic renal failure (CRF) may tolerate hyperkalemia much better than patients with ARF. Potassium greater than 6–6.5 mmol/l requires urgent treatment. Calcium, bicarbonate, and dextrose/insulin buy time prior to dialysis but do not alter the underlying problem. (See Hyperkalaemia p. 133.)

Indications for renal replacement therapy
The management of established renal failure requires renal replacement therapy. Indications for this are shown in Table 6.4.

TABLE 6.4 Indications for renal replacement therapy	
Acute	**Within 24 hours**
K+ > 6.5 mmol/l	Urea > 40–50 mmol/l and rising**
pH < 7.2, deterioration of clinical state	Creatinine > 400 umol/l and rising**
Fluid overload/pulmonary oedema	Hypercatabolism, severe sepsis
**These are nominal values only which are a guide to the probable need for dialysis in acute phase. If values plateau and the patient is passing adequate volumes of urine then consider delaying dialysis: adequate recovery may forestall the need. Patients in chronic renal failure will tolerate higher values.	

Warning! Before commencing renal replacement therapy check hepatitis serology – there is a risk of cross-infection to staff and patients.

Which mode of renal replacement therapy?

Patients with chronic renal failure who require long-term renal replacement therapy usually undergo intermittent haemodialysis two or three times a week or alternatively receive long-term peritoneal dialysis. These modes are usually innapropriate for patients in intensive care. Intermittent haemodialysis is associated with significant haemodynamic instability in sick patients while peritoneal dialysis may be unable to control the biochemistry in the hypercatabolic patient. In addition the peritoneal route is contraindicated in the presence of intraabdominal sepsis.

Continuous haemofiltration or haemodiafiltration systems are, therefore, usually preferred. Such systems allow more gradual correction of biochemical abnormalities and removal of fluid. An additional benefit of filtration is the potential removal of so-called inflammatory middle molecules, toxins and cytokines which may be involved in shock states. These systems can also be used outside specialist renal dialysis centres. (See Peritoneal dialysis below.)

Continuous veno–venous haemofiltration (Fig. 6.1)

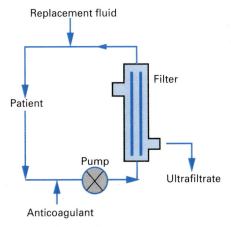

Fig. 6.1 Continuous veno–venous haemofiltration.

When using a haemofiltration system (Fig. 6.1), the patient is connected to an extracorporeal circuit via a double lumen central venous line. Blood is pumped around the circuit, containing a filter which allows plasma water, electrolytes and small molecular weight molecules to pass through down a pressure gradient. The filtrate is discarded and replaced by a balanced electrolyte solution. Overall negative fluid balance can be achieved by replacing less fluid than is removed. Older systems require hourly measurement and adjustment of outputs and fluid replacement. Newer systems are fully automated.

Continuous veno–venous haemodiafiltration (Fig. 6.2)

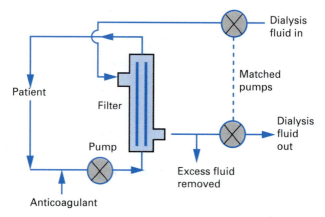

Fig. 6.2 Continuous veno–venous haemodiafiltration.

In continuous haemodiafiltration (Fig. 6.2), dialysis fluid is passed over the filter membrane in a counter current manner. Fluids, electrolytes and small products can move in both directions across the filter depending on both the hydrostatic pressure, ionic binding and osmotic gradients. Overall creatinine clearance is greatly improved compared with haemofiltration alone.

In this system, provided the volume of dialysis fluid passing from the system matches the volume of dialysis fluid passing in, there is no net gain or loss of fluid to the patient. (There is no need to replace fluids in this system.) Fluid volume can be removed from the patient through a side channel on the dialysis exit limb. This is generally controlled by a volumetric pump and rates of up to 200 ml/hour can be achieved. Settings on the machine will vary according to different manufacturers' specification. You should seek advice, or follow your local protocol.

Anticoagulant

In all systems where blood passes through an extracorporeal circuit, anticoagulation is needed to prevent clotting. All patients except those with a severe coagulopathy require anticoagulation. Typical regimens are heparin 1000 units loading dose then 100–500 units/hour or prostacycline 5ng/kg/minute. Infusions are run directly into the dialysis circuit. Excessive anticoagulation can result in bleeding problems. A coagulation screen (APTT) should be performed regularly and the anticoagulant regimen adjusted as necessary.

Problems associated with renal replacement therapy

Complications of renal replacement therapy
Hypotension
Arrhythmias
Haemorrhage
Errors of fluid balance
Line infection
Rise in ICP
Air embolism

It is common to see a fall in blood pressure, cardiac output, and oxygenation when blood enters any extracorporeal circuit. Simplistically this is explained by fluid shifts, haemodilution, and complement/cytokine activation from blood in the dialysis circuit. Hypotension generally responds to simple fluid loading but may require vasopressors/inotropes. Also consider reducing the rate of fluid removal by the system.

Rapid correction of fluid status and biochemistry may cause problems, the so-called dialysis disequilibration syndrome. It is particularly important to avoid this in patients with brain injury in which rapid fluid shifts may acutely worsen cerebral oedema.

Peritoneal dialysis

Peritoneal dialysis is widely used in ARF in small children where adequate vascular access is difficult. In adult intensive care patients, intraabdominal pathology is common making peritoneal dialysis impractical. In septic, catabolic patients it is often impossible to adequately control fluid balance and biochemistry by peritoneal dialysis. Fluid in the peritoneum may result in diaphragmatic splinting. This may impair respiration in the spontaneously breathing patient, and may delay weaning from artificial ventilation in those who are ventilated. Peritoneal dialysis is, therefore, not commonly used in adult intensive care.

Advantages of peritoneal dialysis
Little cardiovascular instability
No need for anticoagulation
Minimal effects on gas exchange in lung

Normal course of established ARF

Most cases of acute renal failure in intensive care patients are due to ATN. The normal course of this condition is spontaneous recovery although urine output does not usually improve until the underlying pathology has resolved. Oliguria (10–30 ml urine per hour, not anuria which is characteristic of obstruction) with a failure to concentrate urine persists for days or weeks followed by gradual recovery of urine output. A diuretic phase may follow. Eventually, there is complete recovery of renal function. The diuretic phase may produce large volumes of dilute urine, which may require replacement. Measure electrolyte losses in the urine to guide this.

High output (non-oliguric) renal failure

This is characterized by rising serum urea and creatinine despite adequate urine volumes. Urine biochemistry demonstrates a failure to concentrate urine. Indications for dialysis are as for oliguric renal failure but there are generally less problems with high potassium and fluid overload. Non-oliguric renal failure is said to have a better outcome than oliguric renal failure.

MANAGEMENT OF CHRONIC RENAL FAILURE (CRF)

Patients with CRF present to the ICU with intercurrent disease. The principles for managing these patients are very similar to those for managing patients with ARF. However, patients with CRF have a number of other, specific, problems.

Problems in CRF

Anaemia
Bone disease
Limited fluid tolerance
Hypertension
Accelerated CVS disease
Vascular access

Patients with CRF are invariably anaemic, but are generally well compensated (may be on erythropoetin, EPO). In the intensive care setting, the need for transfusion will depend on the overall clinical picture and the need for increased oxygen delivery. Hb less than 8 g/dl is a reasonable threshold for transfusion.

Patients with CRF who survive intensive care, will need to return to long-term dialysis. This will require long term AV access. It is important to minimize the number of arterial or venous punctures made. Try to preserve existing sites of vascular access. Take care with AV fistulae: avoid any damage by local pressure or inadequate perfusion. Avoid the subclavian vein on the side of the fistula due to risk of bleeding from vein puncture (arterialized high pressure vessel), and risk of late vein stenosis blocking fistula. Radial artery lines may be best avoided in such cases.

PRESCRIBING IN RENAL FAILURE

Many drugs or their metabolites are predictably nephrotoxic or have the potential to accumulate in renal failure. Renal failure may alter both pharmacokinetics (what the body does to the drug) and pharmacodynamics (what the drug does to the body). This is a large and evolving field, particulary with newer drugs. Consult British National Formulary (BNF). If you are in any doubt, limit yourself to those drugs whose pharmacology is known to you, and seek advice from pharmacist.

Commonly used drugs which impair renal function

- ACE inhibitors
- Aminoglycosides
- NSAIDs
- Cyclosporin
- X-ray contrast media
- Amphotericin
- Cancer chemotherapy drugs

The risks and benefits of starting or continuing such drugs need to be assessed on a daily basis. Consider alternative agents, e.g. fluconazole is an alternative to amphotericin, though it is ineffective against *Aspergillus* and some *Candida* species. Liposomal preparations of amphotericin may reduce its renal toxicity. NSAIDs are usually avoided in at-risk patients, although their effects are usually reversible in the short term.

Drugs cleared by dialysis

Drug clearance is dependant on molecular size, charge, volume of distribution, and water solubility. In general non-ionized drugs with high fat solubility and large volume of distribution will not be cleared efficiently by dialysis (e.g. CNS acting sedative and analgesic drugs).

Opioids

The morphine metabolites (morphine 3 glucuronide and morphine 6 glucuronide) are both active and accumulate in renal failure. It is reasonable to give morphine derivatives as small intermittent intravenous injections but avoid infusing them over long time periods. Pethidine is metabolized to norpethidine which accumulates and may produce cerebral excitation and fits. Phenoperidine is metabolized to pethidine and, therefore, can cause the same problem. Fentanyl/alfentanil accumulate less and may be used for continuous infusions.

Benzodiazepines

The two most commonly used benzodiazepines are midazolam and diazepam. The excretion of midazolam is primarily renal, while diazepam is metabolized by the liver. There are, however, active metabolites of diazepam which are renally excreted, therefore, both drugs have a tendency to accumulate when given as infusions, or as repeated bolus doses, to patients with renal failure.

Muscle relaxants

Muscle relaxants have a tendency to accumulate in renal failure. Atracurium and its isomer cis-atracurium undergo spontaneous (non-metabolic) degradation at body pH and temperature and are the best choice. Vecuronium is an alternative. All three of these drugs demonstrate relative cardiac stability, with minimal release of histamine. Very few other muscle relaxants should be considered. (See Sedation and analgesia p. 24.)

Aminoglycosides

The clearance of aminoglycosides is reduced in renal failure, and high levels are both nephrotoxic and cause deafness if maintained over time. Reduce the dosage/frequency and monitor levels. (See Appendix, p. 267.)

Penicillins

Penicillins accumulate in renal failure and produce seizures at high concentrations. If on high doses consider reduction after loading doses. Carbipenems, cephalosporins and other antibiotics may also need dose reduction in renal failure. Seek advice.

Digoxin

Digoxin is a very unpredictable drug in renal failure. Levels may be substantially elevated compared with healthy patients. It is cleared to a very variable extent by dialysis. It may be safer and more effective to choose a suitable alternative: consider amiodarone or other agents.

PLASMA EXCHANGE

Simplistically plasma exchange works by removing plasma which contains immune proteins. The plasma is typically replaced by 4.5% albumin solution or FFP. There are a number of established indications and it is occasionally used in ICU patients. In general, for acute disease, benefit is only seen if performed in the first few days after presentation.

Indications for plasma exchange

Established indications include:
Guillain–Barré syndrome
Myasthenia gravis
Systemic lupus erythematosis
Other vasculitis (e.g. Goodpasture's syndrome)
Thrombotic thrombocytopenic purpura

Speculative uses include:
Severe sepsis
Pancreatitis

Typically in an adult a 40–50 ml/kg plasma exchange is performed daily (or alternate days) over 5–7 days using an extracorporeal circuit as in dialysis/haemofiltration. The problems associated with plasma exchange are similar to haemodialyis, i.e. hypotension, anticoagulation, fluid shifts, deterioration in oxygenation. Seek expert help and advice. Plasma exchange is generally performed by the blood transfusion service, or renal medicine.

In some inflammatory conditions (e.g. Guillain–Barré syndrome) immunoglobulin solutions may be given as an alternative to plasma exchange. (See Guillain–Barré syndrome p. 187.)

METABOLIC, ENDOCRINE & DRUG ABUSE PROBLEMS

INTRODUCTION

Metabolic and endocrine disturbance is common in the ICU. This may be the primary presenting condition of the patient or may be the result of the complexities of fluid management and/or the effects of prescribed or illicit drug use.

Some typical electrolyte disturbances seen on intensive care are discussed below. Long lists of possible causes have been deliberately omitted. In general aim for slow correction of most abnormalities over a 24–48 hour period to avoid major fluid shifts.

SODIUM

Hyponatraemia

TABLE 7.1 Causes of hyponatraemia

Excess water intake	Hypotonic fluids
	TURP syndrome
Reduced free water clearance	Stress response with raised ADH
	Renal impairment
	Cardiac failure
	Syndrome of inappropriate ADH
Loss of body sodium	GI tract losses
	Renal losses including diuretic therapy
	Adrenal insufficiency
	Hyperpyrexia & sweating

Plasma sodium represents the balance between extra cellular fluid (ECF) volume and sodium. Hyponatraemia is usually due to an excess of fluid (not sodium loss). This is most frequently the result of excessive use of hypotonic intravenous fluids. Treatment is not usually necessary unless the serum sodium is below 130 mmol/litre. Serum sodium below 120 mmol/l may be associated with altered concious level and fits. Consider the underlying cause.

● Change maintenance fluids to 0.9% saline.
● Reduce fluid input.
● If oliguric, consider the need for renal replacement therapy to remove excess fluid.

Warning! In severe cases rapid correction of hyponatraemia can cause pontine myelinolysis. It is recommended that sodium should not rise more than 2 mmol/l per hour and by not more than 12 mmol/l in 24 hours, to achieve a plasma sodium level between 120–130 mmol/l. Do not use hypertonic saline to correct hyponatraemia unless recommended by senior staff.

Excessive antidiuretic hormone (ADH) secretion

This is a cause of dilutional hyponatraemia due to reduced free water clearance. It is most commonly seen as part of the syndrome of inappropriate ADH secretion (SIADH), which may accompany the neuroendocrine stress response to trauma, surgery, and critical illness. Ectopic ADH secretion by tumours may produce a similar picture. Oliguria is accompanied by increased urine osmolality (>500 mosmol/l) and reduced plasma osmolality (<280 mosmol/l). Fluid restriction and a trial of diuretic therapy may be warranted.

Hyponatraemia due to sodium loss

Significant sodium depletion is associated with a reduction in ECF volume. This stimulates the release of aldosterone and causes the kidneys to retain salt and water and lose potassium. Urinary osmolality is raised and urinary sodium is low, less than 10 mmol/l (unless there is an intrinsic renal problem or use of diuretics).

● Replace sodium and ECF with isotonic saline solutions.

Pseudohyponatraemia

Electrolytes are present and measured only in the aqueous phase of plasma but the concentration is expressed according to the total plasma volume. If there is a raised lipid or protein content in the plasma this can produce a spurious result.

Hypernatraemia

High serum sodium generally represents free water depletion. This is generally associated with a raised urea (without rise in creatinine), and an increased plasma osmolality (>290 mosmol/l).

● Review fluid balance regime.
● Give additional free water as 5% dextrose (for example 1 litre over 6–12 hours) or water via NG. Consider diluting enteral feeds with sterile water. (See Neurogenic diabetes insipidus, p. 176.)

POTASSIUM

Hyperkalaemia

Causes of hyperkalaemia

Spurious (recheck result)
Iatrogenic (excess administration)
Renal failure
Addison's disease
Acidosis
Muscle injury (including suxamethonium, crush injury, compartment syndrome)
Cell death (including haemolysis, chemotherapy)

ECG changes may include peaked T waves, broad QRS complexes and conduction defects. Asystole may occur. Urgent treatment should be given to correct the potassium and resolve the underlying cause.

● 10 ml of 10% calcium chloride slow IV bolus. This will prevent any immediate life threatening arrhythmia.
● 50 ml of 50% dextrose plus 10 units of short acting insulin IV (e.g. Actrapid).
● 50 ml of 8.4% bicarbonate. Particularly useful if a metabolic acidosis is present.
● Consider the need for urgent haemodialysis.

Hypokalaemia

Causes of hypokalaemia

Diarrhoea & vomiting
Nasogastric aspirates
Urinary losses (diuretics)
Dextrose & insulin
β agonists
Hypomagnesaemia

Hypokalaemia is relatively common in the ICU. ECG changes may include ST depression, flattening of the T wave and prominent U wave. If severe (<2 mmol/l), cardiac arrhythmias may occur including supraventricular and ventricular extrasystoles and tachycardia and ventricular fibrillation. Correction is by the addition of adequate K^+ supplements to maintenance fluids. If arrhythmias occur more rapid correction may be required.

● Give 20 mmol of K^+ in 20–50 ml of saline over half an hour via a central line. Repeat as necessary. Monitor the ECG during infusion.

CALCIUM

Bear in mind that most laboratories measure total calcium, both bound and unbound fractions. The unbound fraction (ionized Ca^{2+}) which is the physiologically active component, varies with the albumin concentration. Therefore, look at the corrected figure which takes account of protein binding. Alternatively many blood gas analyzers now measure ionized Ca^{2+} directly. The normal range for this is 0.85–1.4 mmol/l.

Hypocalcaemia
Hypocalcaemia is common on the ICU. Typical causes are shown.

Causes of hypocalcaemia
Large volume blood transfusion
Generalized failure of Ca^{2+} homeostasis in severe sepsis
Pancreatitis
Secondary to phosphate accumulation in renal failure
Parathyroid damage after head & neck surgery

Hypocalcemia causes depressed cardiac function, loss of vasomotor tone, muscle weakness, paraesthesia, and tetany.

● Give 10 ml of 10% calcium chloride slow IV bolus.
● If beneficial, consider slow infusion.

In the case of hypocalcaemia secondary to phosphate accumulation there are risks of calcium-phosphate deposition in tissues with over-zealous calcium administration.

 Warning! In cases of refractory shock unresponsive to other drugs calcium may be effective.

Hypercalcaemia

This occurs less commonly and is generally due to an underlying disease process. Symptoms include GI disturbance, confusion, and polyuria. Treatment is by rehydration and the use of calcium binding agents.

Causes of hypercalcaemia
Iatrogenic
Hyperparathyroidism
Malignancy
Sarcoidosis

● Give 0.9% saline to rehydrate the patient. Check plasma osmolality is within the normal range (280–290 mosmol/l).
● Forced diuresis may be used to aid excretion. Frusemide is administered and the urine output replaced with alternating 0.9% saline and 5% dextrose.
● Calcitonin 4 µg/kg s.c. 12 hourly. Calcitonin reduces the rate of calcium and phosphate release from the bones. It is useful in patients with hypercalcaemia associated with malignancy and generally reduces the calcium level within 2 hours.
● Biphosphonates: e.g. disodium etidronate 7.5 mg/kg IV over 4 hours daily for 3 days. These also reduce release of calcium from bones but generally take a few days to achieve maximum effect.
● Corticosteroids may be useful in hypercalcaemia associated with sarcoidosis/ malignancy.

PHOSPHATE

Hypophosphataemia

This is common in the ICU. It is typically multifactorial due to reduced intake (particularly patients on TPN), redistribution and increased losses (especially patients on renal replacement therapy). Hypophosphataemia causes muscle weakness and subsequent difficulty in weaning from ventilators. It also causes failure of many metabolic processes and, if severe, results in depressed conscious level and seizures. It is questionable at what level replacement should occur (<0.8 mmol/l). In most cases as the patient improves so phosphate balance returns. Give intravenous supplements in the form of sodium or potassium phosphate.

● 30–60 mmol phosphate over 24 hours. Diluted in 100–500 ml 5% dextrose.

Hyperphosphataemia

Hyperphosphataemia is generally caused by excessive intake, or decreased excretion, e.g. renal failure. Maintain adequate hydration with 5% dextrose and consider the need for haemofiltration or haemodialysis.

MAGNESIUM

Hypomagnesaemia

Magnesium is the second commonest intracellular cation and as such serum levels are a poor guide to the need for replacement. Serum magnesium (normally > 0.7 mmol/l) is, however, frequently depleted in critical illness and there is growing evidence that magnesium supplementation improves outcome.

Causes of hypomagnesaemia
Diuretics
Insulin
Gastrointestinal tract losses
Parenteral nutrition

Hypomagnesaemia is usually asymptomatic but can give rise to muscle weakness and cardiac arrhythmias. (Hypomagnesaemia exacerbates the effects of hypokalaemia). The treatment is by magnesium supplementation.

● 10 mmol magnesium sulphate IV over half an hour. Followed by 50–100 mmol over 24 hours.

Magnesium can also been used for the control of seizure activity in eclampsia and for control of cardiac arrhythmias particularly supraventricular tachycardia. (See Disturbance of cardiac rhythm p. 57 and Obstetric patient p. 221.)

Hypermagnesaemia

This is less common and generally results from excessive administration particularly in the presence of renal failure. Cardiac conduction may be impaired with prolongation of the PR interval and broadening of the QRS complexes. At extreme levels this may result in cardiac arrest.

- 10 ml calcium chloride IV will temporarily improve cardiac conduction.
- Consider the need for urgent haemofiltration or haemodialysis.

ALBUMIN

Low serum albumin is common in critically ill patients. Albumin is important to maintain colloid oncotic pressure, as a binding protein for drugs and other substances. The threshold for replacing albumin losses is contentious. In many cases low albumin should be considered as a marker of disease severity rather than a problem in its own right. Most clinicians give albumin when the serum concentration is less than 20 g/l or when there are continuing losses.

Causes of hypoalbuminaemia

Malnutrition
Impaired protein synthesis (liver disease)
Increased losses: capillary leakage/renal disease
Inappropriate fluid replacement

Albumin comes in two solutions and is relatively expensive compared to other synthetic colloids.

- 4.5% albumin (contains Na^+ 140 mmol/l). Typically 250–500 ml used for volume replacement purposes.
- 20% albumin (contains Na^+ 60 mmol/l). Typically 100–200 ml used to raise colloid oncotic pressure.

20% albumin raises the plasma oncotic pressure and expands the intravascular space by drawing fluid in from the extravascular spaces. It, therefore, typically expands intravascular volume by factor of $5 \times$ the volume given. It may, therefore, be used often in association with diuretics in an attempt to correct oedema secondary to severe hypoalbuminaemia and may be used in the nephrotic syndrome to replace protein losses.

METABOLIC ACIDOSIS

(See Interpretation of blood gases/Sepsis, p. 76 and 201.)
Metabolic acidosis is common in intensive care. The causes are shown in Table 7.2. The effects of acidosis are increased respiratory drive (unless sedated/paralysed), and at low pH <7.2 reduced cardiac output, and reduced response to inotropes. Hydrogen ions move into cells and K^+ moves out in an attempt to buffer the acidosis and so hyperkalaemia may occur. Treatment depends on the severity, underlying cause and speed of response to interventions.

TABLE 7.2 Causes of metabolic acidosis

Accumulation of H^+	Loss bicarbonate
Ketoacidosis	Vomiting or diarrhoea
Lactic acidosis (shock & tissue ischaemia)	Small bowel fistula
ARF	Renal tubular acidosis
Salicylate poisoning	

● Treat the underlying cause. (See lactic acidosis below and diabetic ketoacidosis, p. 140.)

● If pH < 7.1 or the patient's clinical condition is deteriorating then give 50 ml 8.4% (50 mmol) sodium bicarbonate IV. Check blood gases and repeat as necessary.

Alternatively calculate the dose of bicarbonate as follows; again then check blood gases and repeat as necessary.

$$\text{Sodium bicarbonate} = \frac{1}{2} \times \frac{base\ deficit\ (mmol/l) \times weight\ (kg)}{3}$$

Warning! There are disadvantages to using sodium bicarbonate, including the large sodium load and the theoretical risk of worsening the intracellular acidosis. Therefore, only use if the pH < 7.2 in an inotrope resistant hypotensive patient.

There are a number of other alkalizing solutions commercially available including Tris buffered bicarbonate solution (THAM). Despite theoretical advantages they are not widely used. Ask for advice and seek local guidelines in your unit.

Measurement of lactate

Lactate measurements are increasingly available from blood gas analysers. There is considerable argument as to its value. Whole body lactate can be estimated from a central venous or arterial sample. Raised lactate (> 2 mmol/l) implies anaerobic metabolism and is seen in shock states. This usually corrects with adequate resuscitation. Failure to do so implies critically ischaemic or dead tissue.

Lactic acidosis

Type A

This is the commonest type of metabolic acidosis seen in the ICU and is due to inadequate delivery of oxygen to the tissue. The tissues, therefore, start anaerobic metabolism and produce lactate. This may arise as a result of cardiorespiratory arrest or from inadequate tissue perfusion as seen in shock states.

- Restore adequate oxgen delivery and tissue perfusion. This will generally require IPPV, oxygen and invasive monitoring of cardiac output and filling pressures (PA catheter) with the appropriate use of fluids and inotropes.
- Give bicarbonate as above if necessary.
- Early haemofiltration if renal failure supervenes.

Type B
This is uncommon and is due to the accumulation of lactate without evidence of tissue hypoxia. It may be precipitated by drugs, ingestion of ethanol or methanol, liver failure, and some hereditary disorders.

- Treat underlying condition if possible.
- Give bicarbonate to correct the acidosis. Large amounts may be necessary.
- Consider the need for renal support.

METABOLIC ALKALOSIS

This is relatively uncommon and is due either to the loss of acid (e.g. from vomiting of gastric contents), or from the excessive administration of alkali (e.g. sodium bicarbonate). The metabolism of citrate (anticoagulant in transfused blood) may also produce metabolic alkalosis. (See Fulminant hepatic failure p. 111). Significant potassium loss alone (e.g. diuretic therapy) may also induce metabolic alkalosis.

The classic clinical scenario is seen with protracted vomiting secondary to pyloric stenosis in young children, but it is occasionally seen in adults. Massive losses of fluid, H^+, Cl^- and K^+ leads to a marked alkalosis and shock state. Profound hypoventilation occurs as the body retains CO_2 as a compensatory mechanism. The treatment is aggressive volume replacement with 0.9% saline and added potassium. The use of acidifying agents like HCL or arginine hydrochloride is controversial and usually unnecessary.

GLUCOSE INTOLERANCE

Glucose intolerance is common in elderly patients and some will be on oral hypoglycaemic drugs. These should be stopped and blood sugar monitored. If necessary commence insulin to control hyperglycaemia.

In addition, the stress hormones released in response to critical illness have anti-insulin like effects. When this effect is combined with the effects of exogenous catecholamines used as inotropes, then glucose intolerance and hyperglycaemia is common. This is further compounded by the use of high glucose loads in TPN.

- Start insulin infusion sliding scale. Perfect control is not necessary, indeed it may be impossible to get blood sugar into the normal range in very sick patients. Avoid peaks and troughs in blood sugar.
- Monitor potassium. β agonists and insulin all drive K^+ into cells.

DIABETIC EMERGENCIES

Most are managed on general wards rather than ICU. Occasional patients are moribund or have associated features like sepsis which require intensive care. The source of sepsis may be occult (e.g. renal abscess, best shown on abdominal ultrasound).

Patients with hyperglycaemia or hyperosmolar coma have large deficits of water, sodium, potassium and other electrolytes. Manage these according to basic principles with rehydration, and the control of blood sugar and other metabolic derangements with insulin. Aim for gradual correction of deficits over 24–48 hours. There is a small but definite risk of cerebral oedema which may in part be caused by over rapid correction of electrolyte/fluid abnormalities.

DIABETIC KETOACIDOSIS

Diabetic ketoacidosis is the most common diabetic emergency. It may be the presenting episode in a newly diagnosed diabetic, or may be precipitated in existing diabetic patients by intercurrent illness (increased insulin requirements) or by reduced insulin dosage.

Pathophysiology

There is effectively an inbalance between the hyperglycaemic effects of stress hormones and the hypoglycaemic efects of insulin. Increased hepatic glycogen breakdown and gluconeogensis coupled with reduced cellular uptake of glucose results in hyperglycaemia which in turn leads to polyuria, with loss of water, sodium and potassium. The hormonal changes also result in lipolysis with release of triglycerides and fatty acids which are metabolized by the liver to to ketones which exacerbate the metabolic acidosis.

Clinical features

- Polyuria.
- Polydipsia initially followed by anorexia, nausea and vomiting.
- Ketones on breath.
- Kussmal respiration (hyperventilation in response to metabolic acidosis).
- Abdominal pain and tenderness.
- Severe dehydration and shock.

Management

 Warning! Severe DKA is a life threatening condition frequently occurring in young people. It requires careful management if a satisfactory outcome is to be achieved. The following notes are for guidance but if you have any doubts you should seek senior advice.

● Institute general supportive measures. Give oxygen. If necessary secure the airway and establish ventilation, but beware of cardiovascular collapse! The need for invasive cardiovascular monitoring will depend on the severity of the condition but in general arterial access and CVP lines are minimum. Pulmonary artery catheter and inotropic support may be required in sicker patients. Pass NG tube and urinary catheter.

● Take base line investigations. FBC, urea & electrolytes (sodium and potassium), glucose, and blood gases. Monitor glucose, potassium and arterial blood gases hourly.

● Look for precipitating cause. Send blood for cardiac enzymes, amylase. Send blood, urine and sputum for culture. Get ECG & CXR. Consider abdominal ultrasound. (Abdominal pain is a common feature of DKA.)

● Start IV infusion of 0.9% saline. Give 1 litre in first 1/2 hour and then 1 litre/hour over the next 2 hours, then review. Large volumes may be required to restore circulating volume and urine output. If serum sodium is >150 mmol/l representing significant dehydration consider 0.45% saline.

● Give 10 units of short acting insulin IV. Follow this with an insulin infusion 6–10 units/hour as necessary.

● Monitor the potassium carefully. As the acidosis corrects the potassium will fall. Start potassium infusion 20 mmol/hour as required.

● Acidosis will usually correct as the patient's overall condition improves. If severe metabolic acidosis pH < 7.0 consider bicarbonate (see above).

● When plasma glucose falls to 12–14 mmol/l change fluids to dextrose 4%/saline 0.18% to prevent hypoglycaemia. Continue insulin as a sliding scale infusion and potassium replacement as necessary.

HYPEROSMOLAR NON-KETOTIC STATES

Some diabetic patients may have sufficient residual insulin activity to prevent ketogenesis but not to prevent hyperglycaemia. Polyuria develops which leads to dehydration and hyperosmolar states. Hyperglycaemia, hyperosmolality and hypernatraemia, are typical and these eventually lead to reduced conscious level and seizure activity. Severe dehydration may lead to raised haematocrit and increased risk of thromboembolic disease. Hyperosmolar non-ketotic states are more common in the elderly. It may be precipitated by the stress response to surgery or infection, and the effects of some drugs including: diuretics, phenytoin and glucocorticoids.

Management

● Similar to DKA above.

● Give oxygen. Secure airway and institute ventiltion if necessary. Invasive cardiovascular monitoring. NG tube. Urinary catheter.

● Rehydration. Give colloid (e.g. haemaccel, or gelofusin) to restore circulating volume if shocked. Use 0.9% saline as rehydration fluid (0.45% saline in severe cases). Correct dehydration more slowly than in DKA. Rapid correction may be associated with cerebral oedema and pontine myelinolysis. Typically give 1/2 fluid deficit over 1st 12 hours and remaining deficit over next 12 hours.

● Insulin as in DKA but typically give lower doses, e.g. 3 units/hour.

● Monitor potassium and replace as necessary. Potassium requirements are usually less than for DKA because of the absence of significant acidosis.

HYPOGLYCAEMIA

Hypoglycaemia can be defined as a blood glucose less than 3 mmol/l. It occurs most commonly as a consequence of insulin or oral hypoglycaemic therapy in diabetic patients but may also be associated with some disease states.

Causes of hypoglycaemia
Insulin
Oral hypoglycaemics
Hepatic failure
Adrenal cortical failure
Hypopituitarism
Hypothermia

Management

● Determine the cause and reduce or discontinue hyopoglycaemia agents as appropriate.

● Give 50 ml of 20% dextrose and repeat as necessary. (Boluses of 50% dextrose may be associated with significant disturbances of osmolality and are best avoided.)

● Commence infusion of 10–20% dextrose as necessary to maintain blood sugar. (See Hepatic failure, p. 111.)

ADRENAL DISORDERS

ADRENAL INSUFFICIENCY

Addison's disease (primary adrenal cortical failure) is rare, but should be considered in 'shocked' patients who do not respond to treatment. The typical clinical features are increased pigmentation, weakness, abdominal pain, vomiting, diarrhoea and hypotension. Biochemical findings are hyponatraemia, hyperkalaemia, hypoglycaemia and hypercalcaemia. Aside from general support measures:

● If possible perform a short synacthen test. (Synacthen is an ACTH analogue.) Give synacthen 0.25 mg IM. Measure plasma cortisol before and 30 minutes after. Cortisol level should rise by 2–3 basal level.

● Give steroid replacement therapy. Basal replacement doses hydrocortisone 20 mg am, 10 mg pm. In stress states give larger doses e.g. 100 mg three times daily.

● Consider mineralocorticoid replacement, e.g. fludrocortisone 50–300 µg daily.

Patients on long-term steroid therapy

The significance of pituitary adrenal suppression by longer term steroid therapy is still debatable but most authorities recommend increasing doses of steroids during critical illness. Functional insufficiency of adrenal secretion can occur in severe illness. In refractory shock consider giving replacement doses of hydrocortisone 100 mg tds. Ideally first perform short synacthen test (see above) or random cortisol. The syndrome of adrenal haemorrhage in shock states, classically meningococcal sepsis – the so-called Waterhouse–Friedrichsen syndrome is of debatable significance.

High-dose steroid therapy

High-dose steroid therapy has been tried in shock states but studies tend to show it worsens outcomes. Likewise there is no benefit in traumatic acute brain injury. Steroids have been reported to improve outcomes in some conditions

Conditions in which steroids may be indicated
Asthma, COAD
Pneumocystis pneumonia
Fibroproliferative ARDS
Spinal cord injury
Airway swelling
Cerebral tumours
Meningitis
Autoimmune conditions

Many patients will already be on corticosteroids for management of various disease processes. Equivalent anti-inflammatory doses are hydrocortisone 20 mg = prednisolone 5 mg.

PHAEOCHROMOCYTOMA

This adrenal secretory tumour is a rare cause of hypertension/heart failure. Patients are most likely to been seen in ICU situation in the postoperative period. Patients are typically volume depleted due to catecholamine effects in longer term.

Management

● Preoperatively patients are commenced on α blocking agents. These prevent the hypertensive effects of catecholamines. Relative hypovolaemia is unmasked and fluid loading is required until postural changes in blood pressure are abolished. If tachycardia develops β-blockers may be added only after full α blockade.

● Perioperative dysrhythmias are common and may require magnesium, β- blockers or lignocaine.

● Once the tumour is removed patients may require replacement of catecholamines (e.g. adrenaline or noradrenaline infusion) to maintain blood pressure. These can then be gradually reduced over 2–3 days.

THYROID DYSFUNCTION

The accurate clinical and laboratory assessment of thyroid function is difficult in a normal outpatient/inpatient setting. Laboratory results are tempered by clinical impressions. In the ICU, symptoms of thyroid under/ overactivity are mimicked by many other conditions making diagnosis difficult. Most patients will have reasonably controlled thyroid disease and present with other conditions.

For patients on oral thyroid replacement therapy, the effects of oral thyroxine last 7–10 days so that it is reasonable to wait for gut function to return rather than moving to parenteral preparations which are usually only available as T3. If oral route cannot be used change to T3 (20 μg T3 = 100 μg T4.)

Sick euthyroid syndrome

Thyroid function tests are often abnormal in the critically ill patient. Most sick patients will have results consistent with the so-called sick euthyroid syndrome. The pattern is low T3, low T4, and inappropriately low/normal TSH. This pattern persists until recovery occurs. The current consensus is that it does not reflect clinical hypothyroidism so thyroid replacement therapy is not usually warranted.

Hypothyroidism

Hypothyroidism should be considered in the elderly patient presenting with hypothermia, coma or other non-specific illness. Treat with replacement therapy in the form of oral/parenteral T3, or thyroxine.

Hyperthyroidism

Uncontrolled hyperthyroidism is rarely seen. Management includes antithyroid drugs, e.g. carbimazole, β-blockers and general supportive measures. (See Management of the postoperative patient, p. 212.)

TEMPERATURE CONTROL

Disturbances in temperature regulation are common in ICU. Often the cause will be multifactorial combining abnormalities of central temperature control and environmental causes.

Measurement of temperature

Core temperature measurements may be obtained from the tympanic membrane, nasopharynx, oesophagus, bladder, rectum or from an indwelling pulmonary artery catheter. These reflect the patient's true temperature more reliably than axillary, oral or peripheral temperature measurements.
The core-peripheral temperature gradient gives an indication of the cardiovascular condition of the patient.

HYPERTHERMIA

Hyperthermia is important as a marker for infection or other disease processes. There are a number of causes of hyperthermia.

Causes of hyperthermia
Infection
Systemic inflammatory response syndrome
Adverse reactions to drugs or blood products
Sympathomimetics
Brain injury
Seizures
Malignant hyperthermia*
Heatstroke*
Neurolept malignant syndrome*
(*Rare)

The exact aetiology of hyperthermia is not known for certain. The need to treat a mildly raised temperature of 38–39°C is debatable particulary in sepsis where it has been argued that it is a physiological response to stimulus. Treatment is necessary if the core temperature exceeds 40°C. Prolonged core temperatures of >42°C are associated with a high mortality as all enzyme systems fail.

● Ensure adequate hydration (increased insensible losses).
● Give regular rectal paracetamol. (The use of other NSAIDs is avoided because of risks of renal failure and coagulopathy.)
● Institute passive cooling: wet drapes, ice packs, fans, and gastric peritoneal or bladder lavage with cold fluids.
● If severe hyperpyrexia consider an extracorporeal circuit to actively cool the patient. (Seek senior advice.)

Dantrolene is a muscle relaxant which works distal to the neuromuscular junction. It has an established role in malignant hyperpyrexia, and appears to work after ecstasy ingestion but not other conditions. It, however, has limited side-effects in ventilated patients so should be tried when other measures fail.

● Dantrolene 1 mg/kg bolus repeated every 10 minutes up to 10 mg/kg. (See Malignant hyperpyrexia, p. 220.)

HYPOTHERMIA

Defined as a core temperature below 35°C, hypothermia is associated with a number of adverse effects. These include; arrhythmias, coagulopathy, myocardial depression, vasoconstriction, increased risk of wound infections, prolonged drug clearance and altered acid–base balance.

To avoid missing hypothermia you should always have a high index of suspicion and use a low reading rectal thermometer in patients suspected of being hypothermic.

Common causes of hypothermia

Cold environment in frail elderly patient
Drug overdosage
Cold water immersion
Prolonged surgery with massive fluid/blood losses*
Deliberate cooling during cardiac bypass
Brain protection (neurosurgery)

*In surgical context prevention is better than cure. The use of fluid warming devices, warming blankets and heated humidifiers perioperatively, should help to reduce this problem.

Management

● Exclude other injuries, drug ingestions, myxoedema, pressure necrosis of limbs/rhadomyolysis and renal failure (measure CK). Treat appropriately. (See Trauma, p. 196.)
● Most patients respond to passive slow rewarming with a slow rise in core temperature of abour 1°C per hour. Utilize a warm environment, hot air warming blankets, and warm IV fluids for volume replacement.
● For severely hypothermic patients, core temperature below 32°C, consider more active warming measures such as peritoneal lavage with warm fluids, instillation of warm fluids into the bladder, or partial (femoral–femoral) bypass with a heat exchanger.
● Patients may develop arrythmias on rewarming usually at around 31°C and may need repeated cardioversions. It may, however, be difficult to restore sinus rhythm whilst the patient remains hypothermic. Occasionally under these circumstances profoundly hypothermic patients will be warmed utilising cardiopulmonary bypass.

In profoundly hypothermic patients it may be difficult to determine whether the patient has actually died. This follows cases of patients making a full recovery from prolonged circulatory arrest and deep hypothermia after cold water immersion. Therefore, resuscitation efforts should be continued until the patient approaches normothermia. Remember the maxim, 'you can't be dead until you're warm and dead.' Seek advice.

DRUG OVERDOSE

Overdoses form a major part of acute medical admissions. The majority are not serious but occasionally patients need intensive care. Comatose or unstable patients should not be managed on a general ward in the belief that they are young and fit and will reliably improve over time. Such patients are at risk from complications, in particular pulmonary aspiration and cardiorespiratory arrest.

Potential complications of overdose

Respiratory failure
Aspiration
Dehydration
Cardiovascular instability
Seizures
Hypoxic brain damage
Hypothermia
Pressure sores
Crush syndrome/rhabdomyolysis
Renal damage
Liver failure

MANAGEMENT OF OVERDOSES

Gastric lavage

Gastric lavage may be performed in an attempt to remove tablet debris from the stomach. The indications and contraindications are shown in Table 7.3.

TABLE 7.3 Indications and contraindications for gastric lavage

Indications for lavage	Contraindications for lavage
Paracetamol	Children
Tricyclic antidepressants	Corrosive ingestion
Salicylates	Refusal of consent
Instillation of activated charcoal.	

Gastric lavage is dangerous in the patient who cannot protect his/her airway or cough adequately, because of the risk of pulmonary aspiration. You may, therefore, be called to the A&E department to intubate a patient prior to gastric lavage. Assess the patient for general status, and specifically the ability to cough, gag and maintain his/her airway.

● If the patient is very obtunded it may be possible to intubate without any anaesthetic drugs.
● If not, perform a rapid sequence induction with preoxygenation, cricoid pressure, intravenous induction agent, and suxamethonium.
● Pass the gastric tube under direct vision and then perform lavage. Consider extubation in head down, left lateral position.
● If the patient is not fit to extubate and/or send to the ward, keep the patient intubated and send to ICU. If respiratory effort is feeble it is better to ventilate for a few hours than leave the patient to breath spontaneously with poor tidal volumes. This keeps the lungs expanded and avoids atelectasis while protecting the airway.

Investigations in overdosage

The commonest referral is an unconscious patient who has left a note or is known to have previously taken overdoses. Many patients repeatedly overdose but such patients may develop other causes for their presentation. It is vital to exclude other treatable causes of loss of consciousness, e.g. head injury, intracerebral haemorrhage, hypoglycaemia, meningitis. If in doubt organize CT brain scan.

Aspirin and paracetamol assays are performed in all cases. Alcohol levels can be measured in most centres and may be useful to distinguish intoxication from brain injury. The majority of other assays are unavailable at short notice and are sent to regional centres. Aside from paracetomol it is rare for assays to alter clinical management. Ask the laboratory to save serum in uncertain cases for later analysis and send urine for toxicology screen.

Supportive care

In the majority of cases there is no specific antidote and care is supportive only.

● Support respiration with IPPV. Sedative drugs can usually be avoided and the patient extubated once the concious level improves.
● Monitor ECG and blood pressure. A number of common overdoses are associated with cardiac rhythm disturbances. Avoid central venous access and cardioactive drugs which may trigger a dysrhythmia. Use fluid in the first instance to manage hypotension.
● Monitor body temperature. Hypothermia is common following prolonged unconsciousness and after overdosage with some centrally acting drugs.
● Single short convulsions do not require treatment. Prolonged seizure activity should be treated with diazepam initially followed by phenytoin. (See Brain injury: Seizures, p. 175.)

The typical course is for a patient to require 12–24 hours supportive care before discharge to the ward. All patients who are admitted following deliberate overdose should be seen by a liaison psychiatrist. This is not usually appropriate whilst the patient is on the ICU but should be considered on return to the general ward when the patient is in a fit state to be seen.

MANAGEMENT OF PARTICULAR OVERDOSES

Advice on the management of some common overdoses is given below. There are however a number of regional poisons information centres in the UK which are manned 24 hours a day to provide advice on the management of specific types of overdose and difficult cases (See Table 7.4). You should call these for additional advice.

TABLE 7.4 Regional poisons information centres

Centre	Telephone
Belfast	0123 224 0503
Birmingham	0121 507 5588
	0121 507 5589
Cardiff	0122 270 9901
Dublin	Dublin 837 9964
	Dublin 837 9966
Edinburgh	0131 536 2300
Leeds	0113 243 0715
	0113 292 3547
London	0171 635 9191
	0171 955 5095
Newcastle	0191 232 5131

Sedative and analgesic drugs

Usually they need no specific therapy. Provide assisted ventilation and supportive care until conscious level and respiratory drive improve. Flumazenil and naloxone may be used to confirm the diagnosis in benzodiazepine and opiate overdose but may precipitate seizures, arrhythmias and hypertension – use with care. Do not use these antidotes in an attempt to avoid the need for tracheal intubation, assisted ventilation and ICU admission. They are short acting. If the infusion stops or is pulled out then the patient will rapidly resedate with potentially fatal consequences. Worse still the patient may awaken and self-discharge to collapse once again outside the hospital. (See Intravenous drug abusers, p. 151.)

Tricyclic antidepressants

The antidepressant drugs have sympathomimetic effects which cause the main problems following overdosage.

Effects of tricyclic overdose
Confusion
Seizures
Coma
Dehydration
Tachycardia
Widely dilated pupils
Hyperthermia

Treatment is supportive with resuscitation, control of seizures, and rehydration. Tachyarrythmias are common and may require repeated cardioversions. Antiarrythmic drugs are best avoided, once hypoxia, acidosis, and dehydration are corrected then cardiac rhythm will usually settle to sinus tachycardia. Correction of acidosis with bicarbonate is thought to help by reducing unbound free drug (pKa effect). Typically even after severe problems (e.g. repeated cardioversions) patient will be stable and extubated after 12–24 hours. Often the patient will require no sedation for first few hours. Short acting sedatives/anticonvulsants may be required for a few hours until the patient is stable (propofol infusion ideal).

Paracetamol

Paracetamol poisoning is important as it is the leading cause of hyperacute liver failure in the UK. Relatively low doses of drug may produce fatal liver failure in susceptible patients such as those with preexisting liver disease. In addition the ingestion of other drugs (e.g. anticonvulsants) may increase the toxicity of paracetamol.

The need for treatment is determined by plasma paracetamol concentrations. For those who fall above treatment thresholds, intravenous N-acetylcysteine is an effective antidote if started within 10–12 hours of ingestion. For treatment thresholds and dosage schedules see BNF or contact poisons advice centre.

For those patients who present more than 12 hours after significant ingestion of paracetamol N-acetylcysteine may still be of some benefit. Advice should be obtained from the poisons centre and/or the local liver unit.

Patients who develop liver failure will often have few visible signs of problems for about 48 hours, then will rapidly deteriorate. Established liver failure follows with hepatic encephalopathy, increasing PT time, falling platelet count, jaundice, and renal dysfunction. These patients must be urgently transferred to a regional liver unit for further management, including possible acute transplantation. Do not wait until the patient is moribund with massive advanced multisystem failure. (See Fulminant hepatic failure p. 111.)

Aspirin

The features of salicylate poisoning are hyperventilation, tinnitus, deafness, vasodilatation and sweating. Hyperventilation and sweating result in dehydration. Coma is uncommon but indicates severe overdose. Gastric emptying is delayed and gastric lavage is useful to retrieve tablet debris up to 4 hours after ingestion. For the same reason plasma levels may be misleading if taken within 6 hours.

Blood gases and electrolytes should be monitored. Treatment is by rehydration. If plasma levels are above 500 mg/l (3.6 mmol/l) in adults or 350 mg/l (2.5 mmol/l) in children then forced alkaline diuresis with 1.26% sodium bicarbonate should be used to improve urinary excretion.

In very severe cases, levels above 700 mg/l (5.1 mmol/l) in adults, haemodialysis is the treatment of choice.

Ecstasy

This and other amphetamine derivatives are increasingly seen as a cause of severe toxic reactions. Patients present with signs of sympathetic overactivity similar to tricyclic overdosage above. These reactions appear more idiosyncratic rather than dose related. It is not clear what triggers the response in a particular individual who may have been exposed to the drug before without problems. Hyperpyrexia, rhabdomyolysis, acute renal failure and multiple organ failure are seen in severe cases. Treatment is supportive with cooling measures and dantrolene may be helpful. Seek advice from poisons centre. (See Hyperthermia, p. 145.)

INTRAVENOUS DRUG ABUSERS

The abuse of drugs by all routes is widespread and many patients will require intensive care. This may be due to the effects of drug overdosage, trauma occuring while under the influence of drugs, or as a result of longstanding medical problems from the side-effects of addiction. Pneumonia, sepsis, pancreatitis and other forms of critical illness are all common in this group.

It may not be evident on admission that patients are drug abusers and such information may be unknown to, or not be offered by patients or their friends and relatives. There is a significant risk of such patients being carriers of hepatitis, HIV and other infectious diseases. This highlights the need to use universal precautions at all times when carrying out procedures. (See Universal precautions, p. 226.)

Specific problems include self-neglect, difficult venous access, poor nutritional status, immunocompromise, abscess and right heart endocarditis. Patients may develop symptoms and signs of drug withdrawl. These may be generally managed by the use of standard sedative/analgesic drugs.

ALCOHOL ABUSE

Alcohol (ethanol) is the most commonly used and abused non-prescription drug. Acute alcohol intoxication is a factor in many patients admitted to intensive care, particularly following trauma, whilst chronic abuse is associated with a number of medical problems.

Problems associated with chronic alcohol abuse
Decreased resistance to infection
Severe chest infections are common (TB should be excluded)
Poor nutrition (give B group vitamins)
Alcoholic cardiomyopathy (atrial fibrillation common)
Cirrhosis/liver failure
Gastrointestinal bleeding
Acute confusional states
Autonomic neuropathy
Acute withdrawal states/delerium tremens

In chronic alcoholics withdrawal may result in insomnia, tremor, agitation, and seizures. Delerium tremens, in which patients develop visual hallucinations, is the most serious withdrawal phenomenon. This may occur from 1–5 days following withdrawal and may be life threatening. Treatment comprises adequate sedation together with supportive care.

● Standard ICU sedative regimens (particularly benzodiazepine based) are adequate. Chlormethiazole given by infusion is difficult to titrate, provides a substantial fluid load, and is probably best avoided. (See Sedation & analgesia, p. 24.)

● All chronic alcoholics should receive B vitamin supplements parenterally.

Acute alcohol intoxication

Acute alcohol intoxication produces coma, hypothermia, hypoglycaemia and in severe cases metabolic acidosis. Treatment is supportive including:

● Intubation to protect the airway and ventilation as necessary.
● Gastric lavage.
● Dextrose infusion to correct hypoglycaemia.

HAEMATOLOGY

INTRODUCTION

Haematological problems are common in the ICU. The majority are related to blood loss, the need for large blood transfusions and the development of coagulation disorders. Bone marrow failure and consequent immune suppression are also seen.

BLOOD TRANSFUSION

Critically ill patients require transfusion as a consequence of haemorrhage, the anaemia of chronic disease, marrow suppression, sampling anaemia, and a host of other reasons. There is much debate over the haemoglobin at which transfusion should be instituted. When considering tissue perfusion, haematocrit (%) may be more important: this is approximately given by Hb × 3. Prime considerations are:

● Oxygen carriage and delivery. The oxygen content of blood is given by Hb × SaO_2 × 1.34. Raising haemoglobin is an effective way of improving oxygen content and delivery (See Oxygen delivery and oxygen consumption, p. 46.)
● Myocardial function. Myocardial ischaemia and diastolic dysfunction occur in the stressed heart where haematocrit falls below 0.18. In the presence of coronary artery disease the threshold is 0.24 or higher.
● Rheology. In vitro and probably in vivo, blood viscosity is reduced as Hb falls below 8 g/dl, and rises above 10 g/dl. This may have implications for perfusion of the microcirculation, particularly in critical illness and following vascular surgery.
● Immunology. There is some evidence that transfusion induces a degree of immunosuppression, particularly massive transfusion. This is important following any major surgery, and especially so where surgery has been performed for malignant disease.

Elective postoperative patients tolerate a haemoglobin between 8–11 g/dl. Critically ill patients require a haemoglobin greater than 11 g/dl.

BLOOD PRODUCTS

In the UK, blood is donated by unpaid volunteers, who undergo general health screening, and specific testing for anaemia, hepatitis A,B,C; HIV1,2; syphilis, ABO, RhD grouping, and CMV status. Whole blood is collected into a citrate-based anticoagulant solution (chelating calcium to prevent clotting) and then further separated to yield platelets, fresh frozen plasma (FFP), cryoprecipitate, etc.

● Whole blood is provided in single-donor units. These contain 450 ml of blood with 63 ml anticoagulant, at a haematocrit 0.35–0.45. There are no functional platelets, and factors V, VIII are at 20% normal levels. Other factors and albumin are present at normal levels. Whole blood may be used for replacement of blood loss where clotting factors are also required.

● More usually, red cell concentrates are provided. These comprise 220 ml packed cells with 50–80 ml of an additive solution, often saline-adenine-glucose (SAG) or SAG with mannitol (SAG-M) as a red cell nutrient. The haematocrit is 0.5–0.7. This is the standard product for red cell replacement.

● Red cell concentrate is also available in a leucocyte-depleted form, in which 70–90% of platelets and white cells have been filtered out. This reduces transmission of CMV and causes fewer WBC febrile transfusion reactions.

● Platelets may be single donor or pooled (5–6 donors). 6 units raises platelet count by $20–40 \times 10^9/l$. Platelets should ideally but not necessarily be ABO compatible.

● FFP is single donor. Each unit of 250–500 ml contains both labile and stable factors, including albumin, gamma globulin, fibrinogen, factor VIII. FFP should be ABO compatible. The usual dose is 2–5 units, given where PT > 20s or when more than 5–8 units blood are transfused. After this, PT should be rechecked.

● Cryoprecipitate is provided as 1–6 single donations per pack, suspended in 10–20 ml plasma. Each unit contains fibrinogen 150 mg, VIII 150 IU and fibronectin. 6 units should raise fibrinogen levels by 1 g/l.

Administration

There are local and national variations in product labelling, though the label should always state the nature of the contents (e.g. whole blood, FFP), its storage temperature, expiry date and time, ABO RhD grouping, donation or batch number, and details of the patient against whom it has been cross-matched.

The large majority of transfusion reactions result from the wrong blood being given to the wrong patient.

● Ensure proper labelling of all samples.
● Check recipient identity. You should check the number and name on the bag of blood against both the blood administration form, and the patient's wristband.

Standard giving sets with 170 μm filters are adequate. Avoid microaggregate filters, and never use these when giving platelets. If blood is given through the same set as other fluids, calcium-containing solutions should be avoided. Check for in-bag haemolysis (pink supernatant). Care should be taken to avoid overheating blood. Units of blood opened for greater than 4 hours pose a risk of bacterial infection. Blood should be given through a cannula of at least 18 gauge to avoid haemolysis. Consider the use of a blood warmer.

FLUID RESUSCITATION IN MAJOR HAEMORRHAGE

Key considerations are:

● Ensure adequate vascular access – at least 2×14 gauge peripheral lines or an 8.5 F line such as a Swan–Ganz introducer sheath. This need not necessarily be inserted into a central vein; a peripheral vein may well be easier to cannulate in an emergency, and just as adequate.
● Continue background or maintenance fluids to provide free water, glucose and electrolyte requirements.
● Commence initial volume replacement with a crystalloid or simple colloid such as modified fluid gelatin (e.g. Gelofusine or Haemaccel).
● Continue with packed cells to maintain a haematocrit 0.26–0.32.
● After 5 units of blood, consider changing to whole blood if available and/or giving FFP. Recheck FBC, U&E, clotting or thromboelastogram (TEG).
● Ensure adequate treatment of clotting. In particular, keep the ionized calcium above 0.85 mmol/l. Maintain normothermia with active warming of the patient if necessary.
● After 10 units, recheck clotting. Consider cryoprecipitate, platelets (most likely to help) and further FFP.

RISKS AND COMPLICATIONS

The commonest risk is unavailability of appropriate blood when needed. Three quarters of transfusion-related deaths result from the wrong blood being given. Other risks are relatively minor; recent figures suggest the risk of HIV transmission is around 1 per million donor exposures. Risk of hepatitis C, E, and seronegative hepatitides is probably higher. ARDS and multiple organ failure are also considered to be complications of massive transfusion.

There is a risk of febrile white-cell reactions, hyperkalaemia, haemolyzed transfusions, and bacterial contamination. In major transfusion, there is a risk of reduction in ionized calcium, hypothermia, and transient acidosis.

Acute transfusion reactions are relatively uncommon. They comprise:

● Haemolytic (75% due to ABO incompatibility).
● Anaphylactic (antibodies to IgA in IgA deficient patients).
● Febrile white cell reactions (antibodies to leucocyte antigens).
● Non-cardiogenic pulmonary oedema (antibodies to leucocyte antigens).
● Urticaria (1–2% of transfusions).

Management includes discontinuing the blood and returning the bag to the laboratory, together with a sample of the patient's blood, for further evaluation. Blood cultures should also be sent. Minor transfusion reactions can often be overcome by using a white-cell filter or giving hydrocortisone 100 mg and chlorpheniramine 10 mg. These measures may allow a cautious continuation of transfusion – seek the advice of the haematology department.

JEHOVAH'S WITNESSES

This group of patients have strong religious views which modify their ability to receive blood and blood products. Their religious views should be respected, as failure to do so may constitute an assault. (See Ethical and Legal issues p. 8 and Death and different cultural views p. 13.)

The Jehovah's Witness patient in intensive care may well be unable to give full informed consent. In the case of adults, seek advice from the Jehovah's Witness hospital liaison committee. Individual witnesses have differing views as to what constitutes acceptable transfusion practice. It is important to minimize any potential blood loss, as transfusion is unacceptable. This includes minimizing unnecessary blood sampling. The following are, therefore, broad guidelines only, and may not be completely acceptable to all individuals.

● Blood (red cells, whole blood) FFP, platelets may not be given to Jehovah's Witnesses under any circumstances.

● Predonated blood is generally not acceptable.

● Albumin and cryoprecipitate is accepted by some (but not all) Jehovah's witnesses.

● Factor concentrates: concentrates of specific factors (for example, factor XI, IX, and VII) are generally accepted – seek the advice of your hospital liaison committee.

● Extracorporeal circuits: the majority of Jehovah's Witnesses accept blood which has been passed through an extracorporeal circuit, provided that this blood is maintained in continuity with their circulation at all times. This allows for cardiac surgery (cardiopulmonary bypass) and for renal dialysis. It does not allow for the use of intraoperative cell salvage, except where it is possible to set up the circuit in such a way as to maintain the salvaged blood in continuity with the circulation at all times.

Patients with an anticipated major haemorrhage should, therefore, be managed by supplementation of iron and other haematinics. Erythropoeitin-therapy is acceptable to most Jehovah's Witnesses. A starting dose would be two thousand units per day, given by subcutaneous injection. Side-effects of this treatment include hypertension, headache, and stroke. Not all patients respond to this treatment. Substantially larger doses (up to 50 thousand units a day) have been advocated. Aggressive hypervolaemic haemodilution in the face of anticipated haemorrhage may also be of value. This means that any blood lost will have a lower haematocrit. Techniques such as elective hypotension may further reduce blood loss. Haemoglobin concentrations as low as 4 grams per decilitre may be survivable.

Jehovah's Witnesses developing a clotting disorder pose a special problem. The use of antifibrinolytic drugs (such as aprotinin) is generally acceptable and should be used early on. If there is evidence of endogenous heparins (as evidenced by a prolonged APTT) then consider giving protamine (see below). Management of the coagulopathy will depend on which clotting factors (if any) the individual is prepared to accept.

COAGULATION DISORDERS

Intensive care patients often have clotting disorders. This may be due to a failure of clot formation, failure of clot stabilization, or active breakdown (fibrinolysis). More than one process may be present. Because of this, the advice of a haematologist should generally be sought. The normal coagulation cascade is summarized in Fig. 8.1.

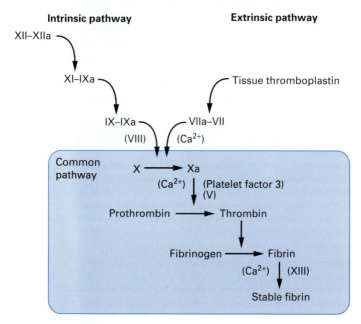

Fig. 8.1 Clotting cascade.

A number of clinical situations contribute to the derangement of the coagulation cascade. Sepsis, multiple system organ failure and related syndromes may reduce hepatic synthetic function of clotting factors. Gastrointestinal absorption of fatsoluble vitamins (A,D,E,K) is reduced. This leads to reduced manufacture of vitamin K dependant factors (II, VII, IX, X, protein C) and coagulopathy. Reduced hepatic reticuloendothelial function permits increased circulating levels of endogenous heparinoids, thus potentiating antithrombin III and inhibiting factors V, X.

Chronic sickness and drugs (ranitidine, heparin and many others) may lead to marrow suppression. Thrombocytopaenia exacerbates impairment of factor X and conversion of prothrombin to thrombin, as well as reducing platelet numbers available for formation of stable clot. In renal failure, the presence of middle molecules may also impair function of platelet surface proteins.

Massive transfusion and vigorous fluid loading can result in 'dilutional coagulopathy'.

Citrate anticoagulants may persist in the circulation for some time, chelating calcium and potentially reducing cardiac contractility. Additionally, some synthetic colloids may impair platelet function (dextrans, hetastarch in particular).

Fibrinolysis may occur as part of a dilutional coagulopathy (see below) or as a consequence of liver disease, where activators of fibrinolysis (t-PA, u-PA) are not cleared from the circulation, while at the same time inhibitors of fibrinolysis (α-2 antiplasmin, α-2 macroglobulin, antiplasmin III) are not synthesized.

Investigations

Platelet count
The normal range is above $100-150 \times 10^9/l$. Platelet counts below $80 \times 10^9/l$ require treatment in the presence of active bleeding. In the absence of active bleeding, platelet counts below $30 \times 10^9/l$ should be treated as there is an incidence of spontaneous intracranial bleeds below this level.

Warning! A normal platelet count does not necessarily imply normal platelet function. Moreover, patients with hypersplenism may exhibit reduced platelet count, but with relatively well-preserved platelet function. Consider a functional test (for example, TEG).

Prothrombin time (PT)
This is normally 12–14 s. Tissue thromboplastin and calcium are added to plasma; the test assays the extrinsic system as well as the common pathway. It is useful as a marker of hepatic synthetic function as well as a guide to anticoagulant therapy (warfarin, discoumarides).

Activated partial thromboplastin time (APTT)
Normally 30–40 s. Phospholipid, kaolin and calcium are added to plasma. This tests the intrinsic and common pathways.

Prolonged PT and APTT are usually due to factor deficiencies, and can be corrected in vitro by the addition of FFP. Failure to correct suggests the presence of inhibitors (e.g. heparin, FDPs).

Thrombin time (TT)
Normal 10–12 s. Thrombin is added to plasma. This assesses the conversion of fibrinogen to fibrin. It is prolonged in the presence of heparin, and activated fibrinolysis (presence of d-dimer or fibrin degradation products (FDPs) which inhibit this conversion).

Fibrinogen levels
Usually greater than 2 g/l; depleted in DIC, dilutional coagulopathy, fibrinolysis, liver failure.

Fibrin degradation products (FDP)
Present only in activated fibrinolysis. Additionally, d-dimer suggests fibrinogenolysis (e.g. DIC).

Thromboelastography (TEG)
This is a dynamic test of clotting and fibrinolysis, which can be used to estimate the need for FFP, cryoprecipitate, platelets or antifibrinolytic therapy. TEG is most frequently used in cardiac surgery and liver transplantation.

Management of coagulopathy
In general, clotting abnormalities should only be treated if there is active bleeding.

● Ensure that the patient is adequately resuscitated. Oxygen, IV access and adequate volume or blood replacement.
● Remember that the commonest cause of bleeding in the postoperative patient is open blood vessels. Surgical causes of bleeding must be excluded before attempting haematological manipulation. Seek surgical advice.
● Other underlying causes of bleeding and coagulopathy should be addressed (sepsis, amniotic fluid embolism, retained products of conception, anticoagulant drugs, aspirin, metabolic derangement, etc.). Do not forget inherited causes, e.g. the haemophilias, although these are rare.
● Perform basic investigations of haemostasis as above. The diagnosis should be clear from a combination of history, examination and the results of these tests.
● If the APTT is prolonged, suspect heparinoids or other inhibitors. The laboratory may be able to repeat the APTT in the presence of a heparinase to help distinguish this. If heparins are present, and you do not know how much heparin has been given, give protamine 50 mg then repeat the APTT. If you know the dose of heparin given, then protamine 2 mg, per mg (100 units) of heparin should provide adequate reversal.
● If the PT and APTT are prolonged in the absence of anticoagulants give FFP which should be administered in 2–4 unit aliquots until PT falls below 20 s. Additionally, if fibrinogen depletion is marked, consider cryoprecipitate 6 units initially.
● If the platelet count is < 80×10^9/l, give 4 units platelets, though more may be required if the count is lower or where the response to transfusion is limited

– for example in DIC. In renal failure, platelet function may be abnormal even if platelet numbers are adequate. Desmopressin (DDAVP) 20 µg as a one-off bolus releases peripheral stores of factor VIII:RAg. This increases platelet 'stickiness' and thereby improves function.

● Check the ionized calcium: if below 0.85 mmol/l, this may contribute to coagulopathy. Give 2.5–10 mmol calcium chloride slowly. **NB** This may result in cardiac rhythm disturbances, particularly if the serum potassium is low. A hypertensive haemodynamic response may also be observed.
(See Hypocalcaemia p. 134.)

● In malabsorption states and liver disease, vitamin K 10 mg can partially correct clotting disorders.

Diffuse intravascular coagulation (DIC)

DIC is a complex process arising as a result of generalized activation of the inflammatory cascade. It involves activation of clotting within the microvasculature, with consequent tissue damage. There is a concomitant consumptive coagulopathy, where normal clotting fails to take place because of depletion of circulating factors. The process is generally accompanied by activated fibrinolysis, with clot instability. The breakdown products of fibrinogen (d-dimer) and fibrin (FDPs) are in themselves anticoagulant, thus adding an extra level of complexity.

The management of DIC presents a therapeutic challenge. Early involvement of your haematologist is essential. The principles of management revolve around treating the underlying cause and adequate replacement therapy with FFP, cryoprecipitate and platelets. Where fibrinolysis (elevated TT, characteristic TEG) is a prominent feature, antifibrinolytic drugs are employed (tranexamic acid 1 g bolus then 300 mg/h by infusion or aprotinin 2 million units bolus followed by 0.5 MU/h). Some units employ antithrombin III in the treatment of this condition – seek advice. There is no role for heparinization.

THE IMMUNOCOMPROMISED PATIENT

Immunocompromised patients are seen increasingly commonly in the ICU. Immune deficiency may be inherited (e.g. severe combined immune defficiency, SCID) or acquired. Most commonly, it is seen in patients with depressed bone marrow function.

Causes of immunocompromise
Cancer chemotherapy
Haematological malignancy
Bone marrow infiltration from any malignant process
Immunosuppressant drugs
HIV infection/AIDS
Chronic illness
Aplastic anaemia (idiosyncratic drug reactions)

Presenting features

Most are referred to ICU with an established diagnosis of immune compromise. Referral is generally precipitated by respiratory failure or sepsis syndrome. Often the time course is short, and the precipitating events may be unclear. Differential diagnosis includes other causes of shock, e.g. hypovolaemia secondary to occult GI haemorrhage. Initial management includes assessment and resuscitation as for any collapsed patient (oxygenation, circulating volume, inotropes, etc.).

General approach

The patient should be transferred to a safe environment where barrier nursing is possible. This is to protect the patient from further risk of infection, as cross-infection with potentially resistant organisms is a major problem in intensive care, and disastrous in the immunocompromised host. (See Infection control, p. 20.)

Some patients (haematological malignancy, chemotherapy) have dedicated long-term lines (Hickman, Portacath, etc.) for feeding or chemotherapy. Avoid accessing these as general-purpose central lines: line infection in these can be problematic. Site a separate central line for general use.

Investigations

Baseline blood count including WBC count may give some clue as to the nature and severity of the immunocompromise. Neutropaenic patients may be assessed by markers of inflammation other than WBC, e.g. C-reactive protein. Once the patient is adequately resuscitated, sources of sepsis must be sought. Clinical history and examination may give a strong clue to this.

● Obvious sites of sepsis should be cultured, abscesses drained, etc.
● Send blood cultures – remember previous multiple broad-spectrum antibiotic therapy may mask growth, predispose to resistant organisms, and further increase the risk of fungal infection.
● Suitable culture media should be used (e.g. bottles with antibiotic binding resins). Alert the microbiology laboratory to this, so they can culture for unusual organisms.
● Protozoal infection – discuss media with laboratory.
● Urine culture.
● Stool culture.
● Serology for viral infection – CMV, herpes, EBV, etc. should be sent.
● *Candida* and *Aspergillus* antigen tests

Pneumonia in immunocompromised patients
(See also Pneumonia, p. 88.)

Impaired gas exchange may be due to SIRS, ARDS or pneumonia. This may be a conventional infection (typical or atypical pneumonia) or an interstitial pneumonitis. Interstitial pneumonitis presents with impaired gas exchange, poor lung compliance and a ground-glass X-ray appearance resembling that of ARDS.

Differential diagnosis
ARDS
Pulmonary oedema
Pneumocystis pneumonia (PCP)
Candida pneumonia
Aspergillus pneumonia
CMV pneumonitis
Tuberculosis
Lymphoma

Diagnosis is helped by bronchoalveolar lavage (BAL). If this is negative on two occasions, bacterial infection and PCP are relatively unlikely. Lung biopsy may be of value in diagnosing CMV, lymphoma and tuberculosis.

Positive diagnosis may be elusive and delayed. It may thus be necessary to start blind therapy. This should be in discussion with the microbiology department. It will generally include a broad-spectrum antibiotic such as piperacillin-tazobactam, and cover for fungal infection (liposomal amphotericin). Some units routinely add in high-dose cotrimoxazole for PCP and antiviral cover such as gancyclovir. These drugs may have toxicity of their own, so give careful thought to their use. For example, both CMV infection and gancyclovir can give rise to marrow suppression – in blind treatment this can confound diagnosis and compound the underlying pathology.

Haematological malignancy

Patients with haematological malignancy represent a tremendous diagnostic and therapeutic challenge in the ICU. A frequent problem is neutropaenia following marrow ablation and transplantation. Very slow recovery of WBC count may occasionally be hastened by administration of granulocyte-colony stimulating factor (GCSF). The combination af haematological malignancy and requirement for IPPV carries a very high mortality especially where the pneumonia remains undiagnosed. (Patients with proven PCP do occasionally survive.) When renal failure is added to this constellation, the mortality is close to 100%.

Aids

Patients with AIDS who develop PCP pneumonia can have a reasonably good prognosis provided multiorgan failure does not supervene. CD4 count is a valuable guide to the likelihood of response to therapy.

Organ transplant recipients

Solid organ transplant recipients no longer require special protection in the ICU during their perioperative course. The same is probably true should they develop opportunistic infections, surgical sepsis or interstitial pneumonias, as their immunosuppression is less severe than those with pathological states. If necessary immunosuppression can be withdrawn. Typically, transplant patients with sepsis can be managed on steroids, their maintenance immunosuppression being reintroduced following recovery or in the event of rejection.

NEUROLOGY

BRAIN INJURY

Introduction

The brain is extremely susceptible to injury from many causes as shown in Table 9.1.

TABLE 9.1 Typical causes and patterns of injury	
Traumatic brain injury	Diffuse axonal injury
	Acute intracerebral haematoma
	Acute subdural haematoma
	Acute extradural haematoma
	(all above may coexist)
	Diffuse swelling
	Contusions (bruising)
Intracranial bleeds	Subarachnoid haemorrhage
	Intracerebral haemorrhage
Cerebrovascular disease	Stroke (haemorrhage/emboli/ thrombotic)
Infection	Meningitis, encephalitis, abscess
Hypoxic/ischaemic brain injury	Asystolic cardiac arrest
	Attempted hanging
	Profound hypotension
	Airway obstruction
	Ventilator disconnection
	Carbon monoxide poisoning
	Prolonged seizures
	Brain retraction
Metabolic	Liver failure
	Hypoglycaemia

Unlike other organs the brain has very limited ability for regeneration. Brain damage starts with the primary insult which may then produce secondary damage, e.g. as a result of swelling.

Practical management revolves around.

● Prevention of primary injury (often too late by time of referral to ICU.
● Stopping the original process of injury.
● Preventing secondary damage from seizures, hypoxia, hypotension, and secondary brain swelling.
● Identifying and treating conditions amenable to surgical intervention. Space occupying lesion (blood clot, tumour, abscess), drainage of hydrocephalus.
● Identifying conditions amenable to medical treatment. Infections (meningitis, encephalitis) and metabolic derangement.

The following information relates, in particular, to traumatic brain injury but the underlying principles are equally valid for brain injury, irrespective of cause.

IMMEDIATE MANAGEMENT

Depending on local policy, you may be asked to assist with the management of head injured patients in the resuscitation room. You should therefore, be familiar with Advanced Trauma Life Support (ATLS) protocols as well as the acute management of the brain injured patient. (See Trauma, p. 190.)

Assessment of patient

The initial assessment includes:

- **A** Airway (with cervical spine control)
- **B** Breathing
- **C** Circulation
- **D** Disability (neurological assessment)
- **E** Exposure (other injuries).

Neurological assessment requires serial documentation of conscious level. In addition any evidence of lateralizing signs (suggesting space-occupying lesion), fundal haemorrhages, papilloedema, and CSF rhinorrhea or ottorrhea should be documented.

The simplest assessment of conscious level utilizes a four point scale:

- **A** <u>A</u>lert
- **V** <u>R</u>esponds to <u>V</u>ocal Stimuli
- **P** <u>R</u>esponds to <u>P</u>ainful Stimuli
- **U** <u>U</u>nresponsive.

The Glasgow Coma Scale (GCS) (Table 9.2) is a more comprehensive neurological assessment which is widely used and has some prognostic value. It should be performed as soon as the patient is stabilized. It is repeated throughout the resuscitation process to identify any deterioration in the patient's condition, which may suggest expanding intracerebral haemotoma or brain swelling. The best motor response is particulary important.

Indications for intubation and assisted ventilation

You should consider early intubation and assisted ventilation in the following circumstances:

- GCS less than 8 or falling rapidly.
- Seizures (continue to treat after muscle relaxants given).
- Hypoxia.
- Hypercarbia (Pa_{CO_2} > 6.5 kPa), or hypocarbia (Pa_{CO_2} < 3.0 kPa).
- Inability to protect airway.
- Significant facial injuries and bleeding (swelling may make intubation very difficult if delayed).
- Major injuries elsewhere especially chest injuries.
- Evidence of shock state (tachycardia, low BP, acidosis, etc.).
- A restless patient who requires transfer to CT.
- Any patient requiring interhospital transfer.

TABLE 9.2 Glasgow coma score (GCS)

Eye opening	
Spontaneously	4
To speech	3
To pain	2
None	1

Best verbal response	
Orientated	5
Confused	4
Inappropriate words	3
Incomprehensible sounds	2
None	1

Best motor response (arms)	
Obeys commands	6
Localization to pain	5
Normal flexion to pain	4
Spastic flexion to pain	3
Extension to pain	2
None	1

Max Score 15. Minimum Score 3. (A modified GCS is used for children under 5 years.)

Intubating brain-injured patients
(See Practical procedures: intubation of the trachea, p. 247.)

Laryngoscopy and intubation is a major stimulus and may produce a significant rise in blood pressure and ICP. Adequate sedation and anaesthesia must be provided to blunt this response in order to avoid potential worsening of the brain injury.

● Establish intravenous access (if not already present). Give volume loading, particularly if haemorrhage and other injuries. Blood or colloid as appropriate. If possible establish direct arterial pressure monitoring.
● Check all intubation equipment, breathing circuits, ventilators and suction etc. Monitor should be available for BP, ECG, Sao_2, & $ETCO_2$.
● Note the baseline pupil size for reference, since this is the only clinical monitor of the brain following anaesthesia and paralysis.
● Assume there is cervical spine injury until proved otherwise. A second person should provide inline immobilization of the neck. (It is useful to use a gum elastic bougie to facilitate intubation without extending the neck.)
● Assume a full stomach and perform rapid sequence induction.
Pre-oxygenate with 100% oxygen. Get an assistant to apply cricoid pressure. Use etomidate if the BP is low, otherwise thiopentone as induction agent. Suxamethonium is used to provide muscle relaxation. Fentanyl 100 μg increments helps to block the hypertensive response to intubation.

Warning! Suxamethonium causes a transient rise in intracranial pressure. However, in the context of the multiply injured patient with brain injury, securing the airway rapidly and safely is essential. Suxamethonium is usually the drug of choice.

● Intubate the patient and pass an orogastric tube, to drain stomach contents. Change to nasogastric only after excluding a base of skull fracture. (There is a risk of a nasogastric tube entering the cranium in the presence of a base of skull fracture.)
● Ventilate to normocapnia or moderate hypoocapnia. (Paco$_2$ 4–4.5 kPa) Monitor the Sao$_2$, ETCO$_2$. Measure direct arterial blood pressure and blood gases as soon as possible. Maintain adequate cerebral perfusion pressure with fluids and/or vasoactive drugs. (see below).
● Maintain paralysis with an atracurium or vecuronium infusion. Maintain sedation with benzodiazepines, propofol and opiates.

Radiological investigations
Plain skull X-rays may be useful in the initial evaluation of patients with mild head injuries, as the presence of a skull fracture greatly increases the risk of subsequent intracerebral haematoma. However, in the severely head injured patient CT scans should not be delayed by taking plain X-rays. Skull fractures are well visualized on CT films.

CT scan
CT scanning is fundamental to the modern management of brain injury. It is essential if brain injury is suspected or cannot be excluded because the patient is already anaesthetized and ventilated. CT scan will:

● Confirm diagnosis, e.g. head injury, subarachnoid bleed, tumour.
● Identify space occupying lesion.
● Direct surgery to site of injury.
● Often be apparently normal in diffuse hypoxic injury.

Warning! CT scans are very dependant on skilled interpretation. Do not make clinical decisions until senior experienced staff have reviewed them. Minor subarachnoid bleeding, mild cerebral oedema, early cerebral infarction, pituitary lesions, and brain-stem lesions are all easily missed.

Multiple injuries in the brain-injured patient
Traumatic brain injury may be an isolated injury but this should never be assumed. The care of the brain injury must proceed alongside the continuing re-evaluation and resuscitation of the other injuries according to ATLS protocols. In particular remember:

- Cervical spine injury (immobilize, X-ray lat. C spine).
- Cardiothoracic trauma (CXR, ± drains).
- Abdominal injuries (diagnostic peritoneal lavage, US, CT, laparotomy).
- Pelvic fractures (X-ray, early external fixation).
- Splint limb injuries (assess neurovascular integrity).

Which injury should take priority?

In the multiply-injured patient with a brain injury priorities must be decided.

- Many brain injuries do not require neurosurgical intervention.
- Any brain injury will be worsened by significant hypoxia or hypotension.

Any injury which compromises the airway, breathing, or circulation takes priority. In particular life threatening bleeding from the chest or abdomen requires immediate surgical intervention and should not be delayed by CT head scan or neurosurgery. In exceptional cases blind burr holes or craniotomy can be performed simultaneously with other surgery and CT scan performed before transfer to ICU.

Warning! The correct course of action will depend upon the circumstances of the case and the local expertise and facilities. However, the death of a patient in the CT scan from a ruptured spleen is a disaster, all the more so if the scan is unremarkable! Only transfer patients when you are sure they are stable. Seek senior help.

Management

On the basis of the CT scan there may be a number of options for the further management of the patient.

- Normal or minimal changes. Stop sedative drugs, allow the patient to wake and reassess neurological state.
- Diffuse, or non-operable injury (diffusely swollen brain). Admit to ICU for further management including monitoring of ICP.
- Space occupying lesion with a mass effect requires urgent neurosurgical referral and craniotomy.

Which patients require referral to specialist neurocentre?

The facilities available in local hospitals for dealing with the head injured patient vary from hospitals with no CT scan, and hospitals with CT scan but no neurosurgery, to hospital centres with all facilities. The decision to transfer a patient will, therefore, be influenced not only by the patient's condition but also the local availability of resources.

Indications for urgent referral to neurosurgical centre
No CT scan available locally
CT scan shows haematoma causing mass effect
Diffuse brain injury with raised ICP
Deteriorating GCS regardless of CT scan appearances
No ICU facilities available locally

Identification of a vacant ICU bedspace should not delay transfer of cases who require urgent CT scan or craniotomy for evacuation of haematoma. Most neurosurgical units adopt an open admission policy, taking all serious injuries for CT scan, and operative intervention where appropriate, regardless of the availability of ICU beds. Once appropriate interventions have been performed, any delay in finding an intensive care bed will not place the patient at further significant risk.

Indications for less urgent transfer include:

- Isolated depressed skull fractures with no neurological deficit.
- Isolated CSF leaks.
- Patients with lesser injuries who fail to improve neurologically over time.

ICU MANAGEMENT OF BRAIN INJURY

There are a number of key concepts which underlie the intensive care management of the brain injured patient.

1. Autoregulation

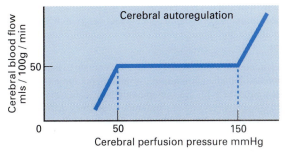

Fig. 9.1 Cerebral autoregulation.

Normally, cerebral blood flow is maintained at a constant level over a range of cerebral perfusion pressures, a process known as autoregulation. Cerebral blood flow is also increased by hypercarbia and hypoxia and reduced by hypocarbia.

In previously hypertensive patients the curve is shifted to right and autoregulation occurs at higher blood pressures. In the brain injured patient autoregulation is often deranged and cerebral blood flow is critically related to cerebral perfusion pressure.

2. Cerebral perfusion pressure (→ Table 9.3)

Cerebral perfusion pressure = Mean arterial BP–Intracranial pressure
$\qquad$ (CPP) $\qquad$ (MABP) $\qquad$ (ICP)

TABLE 9.3 Typical values cerebral perfusion pressure	
Adults	CPP > 60 mmHg
3–12 years	CPP > 50 mmHg
<3 years	CPP > 40 mmHg

3. Intracranial compliance

The skull is effectively a rigid box containing the brain, CSF and blood. If the volume of one of these components is increased, e.g. by the presence of an intracranial haematoma, or cerebral oedema, then the volume of the others must be reduced. Initially CSF is displaced into the spinal canal followed by a reduction in blood volume. Eventually when no further compensation is possible, the ICP will rapidly rise and the brain itself may become displaced and herniate.

GENERAL MANAGEMENT

There is no evidence that specific regimes designed to produce cerebral protection, e.g. the use of barbiturates, or steroids, alter the outcome of brain injured patients. ICU management is based upon maintenance of adequate cerebral perfusion and oxygenation in order to prevent secondary brain damage, and limitation of cerebral oedema and surges in ICP to prevent brain herniation. Other general principles of management are the same as for any patient.

● Maintain adequate sedation and paralysis. Ventilate to maintain adequate oxygenation and initially normocapnia, or mild hypocapnia ($Pa\text{CO}_2$ 4–4.5 kPa).
● Nurse the patient 15–30° head up to ensure adequate venous drainage. Avoid tight tapes to secure endotracheal tube which may occlude jugular veins.
● Establish monitoring. Arterial blood pressure and CVP, urinary catheter, NG tube. Avoid internal jugular routes of cannulation except for jugular bulb cannula. Insertion difficulties may impair cerebral venous drainage and also risk carotid injury. The femoral route may be best choice, to avoid need for head down tilt during insertion.
● Maintenance fluids 0.9% saline (plus K^+) initially. In the past maintenance fluids were restricted, but maintenance of cerebral perfusion is now considered paramount. Hyponatraemia and hyperglycaemia worsens outcome and should be avoided.

● Stress ulcer prophylaxis. Commence enteral feeding as soon as practicable. Otherwise NG sucralfate should be prescribed.

Maintenance of cerebral perfusion pressure (CPP)

Maintain CPP greater than 60 mmHg in adult patients. It may need to be even higher in elderly hypertensive patients (normal autoregulation curve shifted to the right) or if there is evidence of cerebral vasospasm (e.g. in subarachnoid haemorrhage), or evidence of inadequate perfusion (e.g low SjO_2) (See below.)

● Titrate fluid therapy according to CVP. If no improvement or if the patient is haemodynamically unstable consider use of pulmonary artery catheter.
● After adequate fluid resuciation if CPP remains low, use vasopressors, e.g noradrenaline or phenylephrine to increase mean arterial pressure and improve CPP. Adrenaline may be used if invasive monitoring indicates that the primary reason for a low MAP is low CO.

Control of intracranial pressure (ICP)

The measurement of ICP is now routine practice in the management of head injury. It is also being increasingly applied to other conditions where there is likely to be raised ICP, for example, in the management of metabolic conditions such as liver failure. It is used to give an indication of increasing cerebral oedema, the re-accumulation of haematomas, and to calculate CPP.

Normal ICP is less than 10 mmHg and a sustained pressure higher than 20 mmHg is associated with worse outcomes. If ICP is greater than 20–30 mmHg then intervention may be necessary, particularly in the first 24–48 hours. Table 9.4 gives a check list of causes of a raised ICP. Check and exclude measurement errors and avoidable rises before starting treatment.

TABLE 9.4 Management of raised ICP

Problem	Action
ICP accurate?	Reposition, flush and recalibrate device
Inadequate sedation or paralysis	Give bolus of sedation and relaxants Increase infusion rates
Hypoxia or hypercarbia	Check blood gases Alter ventilation appropriately
Inadequate CPP	Give additional fluids Increase vasopressors/inotropes
Venous drainage from head and neck impaired	Check head twisted, tapes too tight Nurse 15–30° head up
Seizures	Often masked by muscle relaxants check CFM trace. Stop/reduce relaxants temporarily
Pyrexia	Give antipyretics Pyrexia increases cerebral oxygen requirements therefore increase oxygen delivery and CPP

If all factors are optimized exclude development or reaccumulation of haematoma. Consider repeat CT scan and seek surgical opinion. Correct any coagulation defects. Other measures to control ICP include:

1st line

● Mannitol 0.5 g/kg over 20 minutes, and/or frusemide 0.5 mg/kg. Any benefit tends to be temporary.
● Moderate hyperventilation to lower Pa_{CO_2}. Keep Pa_{CO_2} >4 kPa. Lower levels may result in excessive cerebral vasoconstriction and may produce areas of ischaemia. Any benefits will tend to disappear over a few hours.
● CSF drainage via external ventricular drain.
● Ensure that adequate CPP is maintained at all times. If there is no response to simple measures, consider further increasing CPP. The benefit of this may not be immediate and may take a few hours.

2nd line

● Thiopentone infusion. 15 mg/kg 1st hour, 8 mg/kg 2nd hour, 5 mg/kg/hour thereafter. Monitor levels over time.
● Decompressive craniotomy. Lobectomy and do not replace bone flap.
● Induced hypothermia.
● Aggressive hyperventilation to Pa_{CO_2} <3 kPa. See note above.

Newer monitoring modalities

There are a number of newer monitoring modalities currently under evaluation in brain injury which you may encounter. These include:

● Jugular bulb oxygen saturation (Sj_{O_2}).
Measuring the saturation in venous blood from the brain gives an indication of the adequacy of oxygen delivery and utilization by the brain. The normal range is 55–75%. Changes are more valuable than isolated values. If Sj_{O_2} is low, consider measures to improve cerebral blood flow, in particular raising CPP.

If the saturation is high then the brain is either hyperaemic or failing to extract oxygen. Barbiturates may be helpful to control ICP in the presence of hyperaemia. In brain death the saturation may approach 100% as the brain ceases to extract oxygen.

● Transcranial doppler (TCD). Gives an estimate of blood flow in individual vessels, e.g. middle cerebral artery.
● Near infrared spectroscopy. Gives an estimate of brain tissue oxygenation by the absorbtion of light by cytochromes.
● Brain tissue PO_2. A miniaturized electrode is placed within or on the surface of the brain to measure tissue PO_2 directly.

COMMON PROBLEMS IN BRAIN INJURY

Widely dilated pupil

Sudden increases in pupil size, particularly if unilateral and non-reactive to light, may be due to stretching of the 3rd cranial nerve and may herald brainstem herniation. This is an indication for urgent repeat CT scan. Dilated pupils may reflect underlying seizure activity. Bilateral fixed dilated pupils are an ominous sign of impending brain death but should not be considered in isolation.

Seizures

Generalized or focal seizures are common with brain injury from any cause. In the complicated ICU patient the distinction between focal and generalized seizures is indistinct and usually of little relevance.Such patients with repeated seizures will almost always be ventilated. The peripheral manifestations of seizures will be masked by the use of muscle relaxants, but their damaging effects on the brain will continue if left untreated.

Cerebral function monitors (CFM) may be used to detect abnormal seizure activity. The simplest of these displays two channels, base line activity (to detect artefacts) and global cerebral electrical activity. Typical traces are shown in Fig.9.2. The 'saw tooth' pattern is typical of seizures.

Newer forms of cerebral function monitors have multiple channels and display the electrical activity of each cerebral hemisphere separately. You should seek advice on the interpretation of these. If in doubt in the paralyzed patient request a formal EEG. Alternatively there is usually little harm in temporarily reducing/stopping muscle relaxants to assess seizure activity; ensure adequate doses of sedative/analgesic drugs first!

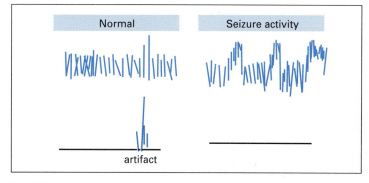

Fig. 9.2 Cerebral function monitoring.

Continued seizure activity increases oxygen requirement of the brain and worsens brain injury Therefore seizures should be treated promptly.

● Exclude any treatable precipitating cause such as hypoxia, hypercarbia, hyperthermia or electrolyte disturbance.

1st line

● IV benzodiazepines e.g. diazepam 5–10 mg or clonazepam as necessary. Large cumulative doses may be needed. Midazolam is also effective.
● IV phenytoin. Loading dose 15 mg/kg. Give 300 mg loading dose over 1 hour and then 1200 mg over next 24 hours. Daily dose 300 mg thereafter. Measure levels over time. May cause disturbances of cardiac rhythm in some patients.
● IV propofol, bolus followed by infusion 200–400 mg/hr may also be effective.

2nd line

● If seizure activity is not controlled additional anticonvulsant agents such as sodium valproate, phenobarbitone, chlormethiazole, paraldehyde or magnesium, may be required. Seek advice and check dose regimens in BNF.
● Consider thiopentone bolus 500 mg over 5 min, followed by infusion 2.5–5 g daily. Check levels over time.

Prophylactic anticonvulsants

Prophylactic anticonvulsants are commonly given in at-risk patients. For example, patients with significant contusions on CT or documented seizures after injury. Phenytoin is the usual drug as it does not produce significant sedation (See doses above.)

Neurogenic diabetes insipidus (DI)

Neurogenic DI results from failure of the posterior pituitary to produce ADH. It may result from either localized damage to the pituitary/hypothalamic area or from diffuse brain injury, as in brain death. It is usually seen in first 24–48 hours postinjury and is manifest as an excessive urine output due to inability to concentrate the urine. Untreated, this results in hypernatraemia.

DI should be considered if urine outputs persist at greater than 300–400 ml/hour in absence of diuretics. Other causes of excessive urine output include excretion of resuscitation fluids, use of dopamine/dopexamine, mannitol and diuretics.

● To confirm the diagnosis check urine/plasma osmolalities. Normal plasma osmolality 286. If increased >310 mosmol/l then urine should be highly concentrated. In this context urine osmolality <500 mosmol/l implies DI.
● Replace urinary losses with 5% dextrose with added K+.
● Give DDAVP 1–2 μg IM or IV as required.

Cardiovascular instability

Haemodynamic instability is common and may be seen in association with neurogenic pulmonary oedema. The importance of an adequate cerebral perfusion pressure has already been stressed. Hypotension may be due to a combination of factors. You should exclude causes such as hypovolaemia, pneumothorax and sepsis.

All patients should have direct arterial pressure and CVP monitoring. In complex cases insert a PA catheter to guide fluids, inotrope, and vasopressor therapy as for any shock state.

Poor pulmonary gas exchange

Respiratory problems are very common in the presence of brain injury and are often the reason for initial ICU admission or delayed discharge. The precise mechanisms are multifactorial but may include inadequate cough and gag reflexes, pulmonary aspiration, chest infection (particularly staphylococcal), pulmonary capillary leak, and depressed immune function. (See nosocomial pneumonia p. 91.)

Most patients with severe brain injury will require a tracheostomy to facilitate airway management for short to medium term care. Neurological function is typically assessed 48–72 hours post injury. Consider early tracheostomy in the seriously brain injured patients. Try to avoid the scenario of repeated extubation, and reintubation and then subsequent tracheostomy. Tracheostomy protects the airway, is more comfortable for the patient, allows early reduction in sedative and analgesic drugs, aids nutrition and mobilization, and allows easier weaning of ventilatory support.

Neurogenic pulmonary oedema

Pulmonary oedema is an unusual but well-recognized complication of brain injury and may accompany catastrophic fatal injury. It may, however, also be seen in patients who subsequently make a full recovery.

In its severest form it is characterized by extreme cardiovascular instability with profuse pink frothy pulmonary oedema. Simplistically, it results from a rapid rise in ICP which produces a catecholamine surge, with subsequent pulmonary hypertension and leakage of pulmonary capillaries. A similar clinical scenario may follow strangulation or acute airway obstruction.

The management is supportive with IPPV, high FiO_2, and PEEP. Diuretics are not usually effective and the volume of fluid leaking into the alveoli and out of the lung may lead to marked hypovolemia. Cardiac instability will often require invasive monitoring with a PA catheter, inotropes and vasopressor therapy. The pulmonary oedema usually settles over time but may develop into severe ARDS. (See ARDS p. 98.)

Cerebrospinal fluid (CSF) leaks

Clear or blood stained fluid from nose or ear may represent a CSF leak which is a feature of injuries to the frontal sinus and base of skull. CSF tests positive for glucose on test strips. In the past antibiotic prophylaxis was popular but most centres have stopped this practice. It is usual to wait about 10 days to see if the leak will cease spontaneously then consider craniotomy and placement of a dural patch.

The irritable brain injured patient

Irritability and restlessness are common in patients with minor brain injury or in the recovery phase of more severe injuries. In the latter there will often be severe movement disorders in the form of extensor spasms. Despite the theoretical risks of masking neurological signs it is often necessary to give sedatives (benzodiazepines) and major tranquillizers (chlorpromazine/haloperidol) to such patients to allow nursing care and prevent further injury. The patient with extensor spasms will need a tracheostomy to stop him/her biting on the endotracheal tube and causing obstruction, and may require very large doses of drugs to settle. Consider nursing such patients on a mattress on the floor to avoid them falling out of bed (cot sides do not always prevent this and increase the height of the fall!).

PREDICTION OF OUTCOME

Outcome following brain injury depends on a number of factors including: the mechanism and severity of the initial injury, subsequent episodes of hypotension, hypoxia or hypercarbia, adequacy of resuscitation, and the presence of other injuries. Age is important, young patients have a substantially better outcome than elderly patients for a given injury. In particular young children may make a good recovery from an apparently devastating injury. There is a wide spectrum from mild to devastating injury. It is relatively easy to predict outcomes at either end of the spectrum but not in between. The passage of time (weeks/months) is essential to assess potential for recovery. Clinicians learn from experience that it is often impossible to predict longer term outcome in any individual patient.

SUBARACHNOID HAEMORRHAGE (SAH)

Patients with sponatenous SAH frequently require intensive care, either early at presentation, after surgery or some time later due to respiratory or other complications.

Patients present with sudden onset of headache, neurological deficit and collapse. Subarachnoid haemorrhage is confirmed by CT scan and or lumbar puncture. The site and appearance of bleeding may suggest an aneurysm or arteriovenous malformation. There are associations with other diseases, e.g. atheromatotus vascular disease, polycystic kidney disease, collagenous/connective tissue disease and other congenital malformations.

Patients can be graded clinically as shown in Table 9.5.
Grading is difficult once the patient is sedated/ventilated. Rebleeding or vasospasm may rapidly worsen neurological state.

TABLE 9.5 Grading of patients with SAH

Grade	Description
0	Unruptured aneurysm
I	Asymptomatic Minimal headache or rigidity
2	Moderate headache & nuchal rigidity No neurological deficit except cranial nerves
3	Drowsiness, confusion, mild focal deficit
4	Stupor, hemiparesis
5	Deep coma, decerebrate rigidity, moribund

Early management

Large intracerebral haematoma may require surgical evacuation (+/− clipping of aneurysm) and intraventricular drainage can be used to decompress the brain and treat hydrocephalus. The timing and indications for subsequent angiography and definitive surgery are controversial. Not all aneurysms or artriovenous malformations are suitable for surgical correction and the role of interventional radiology is increasing.

In operable cases, early surgery reduces the risk of rebleeding, and the development of intercurrent medical problems, but is technically more difficult and increases the risk of vasospasm. Delayed surgery (10–14 days postbleed) is technically easier, carries less risk of vasospasm but increases the risk of bleeding in the intervening period.

The patient's age (increasing risk of cerebrovascular disease and cerebral infarction), preoperative status, and the site of the lesion are important in decisions related to surgery. In general, early angiography and clipping of aneurysms is indicated in the younger patient with milder grade 1–2 signs and aneuryms in anterior cerebral circulation.

ICU management

The management of subarachnoid haemorrhage is essentially no different from other causes of brain injury. Cerebral vasospasm may occur; its exact mechanism is uncertain. In simple terms it is the development of vascular spasm in cerebral arteries which leads to areas of ischaemic infarction. It can be diagnosed by angiography or transcranial doppler.

- Maintenance of cerebral perfusion pressure using fluids and vasopressors is crucial. Aim for mean systemic pressure of 90–100 mmHg. It is not usual to monitor ICP. Vasopressor therapy is usually used and may be required for up to 3 weeks.
- The Ca^{2+} channel blocker nimodipine has been shown to improve neurological outcome. Its effect is thought to be independent of any antispasm action. Its systemic vasodilator effects may worsen CPP and require vasopresor therapy. It is available in oral and IV preparations.

● Cardiac arrhythmias are common in SAH. These do not usually require treatment.

Typically many patients are managed on HDU/ward area. More severe cases may need a period of ventilation in ICU followed by period of weaning and tracheostomy.

HYPOXIC BRAIN INJURY

This problem is most commonly seen following resuscitation from prolonged cardiac arrest. Other causes include:

● Profound hypotension/hypoxaemia from any cause.
● Prolonged seizures.
● Carbon monoxide poisoning.
● Attempted strangulation or hanging.

Patients who are resuscitated following cardiac arrest are usually referred for intensive care because of haemodynamic instability or inadequate respiratory effort. There is no evidence to suggest that periods of elective ventilation, or the use of so-called cerebral protection agents (e.g. barbiturates/steroids) effect neurological outcome. The emphasis should be on prevention of secondary insults.

● Ventilate for 12–24 hours, without sedation if possible, then reassess neurological state. If the patient begins to get agitated then short acting agents, e.g. propofol allow subsequent periodic reassessment of neurology.
● Purposeful or semi-purposeful movements are a good sign and usually herald a full recovery. Absence of respiratory effort, myoclonic jerking and fixed dilated pupils usually indicate severe hypoxic damage and a poor long-term outlook.

A similar scenario is also seen following prolonged hypoglycaemia. This usually follows deliberate overdosage with insulin. (See Management of patients following cardiac arrest p. 73 and Hypoglycaemia p. 142.)

Outcome
The prediction of long-term outcome after hypoxic brain injury is difficult. In the patient who does not awaken, longer term management will depend upon the patient's background health, age, previous wishes (advance directives, etc.). The patient's relatives and family need to be kept aware of the situation and their wishes must also be considered. Unless a consensus is reached regarding withdrawal of active management the patient should be stabilized, weaned off IPPV usually via a tracheostomy, established on enteral feeding and transferred for ward-based care awaiting neurological change over time. When all parties agree that further treatment is futile it is reasonable to wean off assisted ventilation, extubate the trachea, write a 'do not resuscitate' order and await events.

INFECTION

Meningitis

It is rare for adults or children to require intensive care following meningitis. In the case serious enough to warrant intensive care it is advisable to CT scan prior to lumbar puncture (LP) to exclude cerebral oedema and potential risk of coning after LP. In cases of doubt, blind antibiotic therapy is started and LP avoided. Steroids have been shown to reduce longer term neurological sequelae in children with meningitis but their place in adults is less clearcut.

Encephalitis

As for meningitis it is rare for adults or children to require ITU. Occasionally encephalitis needs to be considered as a diagnosis of exclusion in cases of coma. There are characteristic EEG changes with herpes encephalitis. A brain biopsy may be indicated to confirm the diagnosis. Start empirical acyclovir until diagnosis is proved/disproved.

Brain abscess and tumours

Rare causes for ITU admission. High-dose steroids (e.g. dexamethasone) have an established role in space-occupying tumours. Immunosuppressed patients (e.g. HIV) may present with unusual CNS abcesses/meningitis-like toxoplasmosis and cryptosporidiosis.

BRAIN-STEM DEATH

Brain-stem death is caused by irreversible damage to the brain stem, which is the control centre for the autonomic functions of the brain. Its description in 1959 followed the introduction of assisted ventilation in brain injured patients. The intention was to reliably identify hopeless cases who had nothing to gain from further treatment. There have been no verified cases of recovery or long-term survival in patients fulfilling criteria for brain-stem death, as stated in the UK. Brain-stem death is a clinical diagnosis and does not require confirmatory tests such as EEG/angiography in the UK. You will not be expected to diagnose brain-stem death but you should understand the process.

It will usually be clear from clinical bedside observations that brain-stem death has occurred. The typical features of brain-stem herniation are tachycardia and hypertension, followed by bradycardia, hypotension and pupil dilatation. A lack of response to endotracheal suctioning, turning, and mouthcare with fixed dilated pupils suggest the diagnosis of actual or impending brain death. All are performed routinely during nursing care. Formal brain-stem death tests are then used to confirm that brain-stem death has already occurred. It looks unprofessional to do brain-death tests and then find that the patient is not brain dead after all!

Preconditions

 Warning! The preconditions for the diagnosis of brain-stem death are absolutely fundamental and must be satisfied before consideration of the diagnosis.

These are:

- Known cause of brain damage, e.g. trauma, intracerebral haemorrhage.
- Absence of any CNS depressant drugs. Sufficient time must have lapsed to be certain that centrally acting drugs have been metabolized and cleared. Beware of active metabolites which may have long half-lives.
- Absence of neuromuscular blocking drugs. Use a nerve stimulator.
- Normothermia (core temp > 35.5°C).
- Normal metabolic and endocrine state. No significant electrolyte or blood glucose disturbance.

Active measures to maintain blood pressure, temperature, and normal electrolytes are required if the patient is to fulfil preconditions, and to be potentially suitable for organ donation. This may require fluids, inotropes (adrenaline first choice), vasopressors and DDAVP for the hours prior to tests (often overnight). Replacement of the large urine volumes seen with diabetes insipidus (see below) with isotonic saline or synthetic colloid solutions will lead to progressive hypernatremia. Use DDAVP and fluid replacement with dextrose solutions to avoid this.

Brain-stem death tests

The tests are carried out by two doctors who are five years post registration. This is usually two consultants or one consultant and one senior trainee. At least one of the doctors should have been responsible for the patient during his/her admission and neither should be associated with the transplant services. The tests may be performed together or separately, providing each doctor satisfies himself/herself of the results. The tests are repeated at a suitable interval to confirm the findings and the time of death is taken to be the time of completion of the second set of tests. Occasionaly families will request to observe the tests being done. This is acceptable providing they understand the nature of the tests. The whole process of testing, counselling the family and explaining the concept of brain death and organ donation is of necessity, extremely time consuming.

Most hospital have preprinted documentation for brain-stem death tests and organ donation. The tests required are listed in Table 9.6.

TABLE 9.6 Brain-stem death tests	
Test	**Brain-stem function (cranial nerve)**
Pupil light reflex	II, III
Corneal reflex	V, VII.
Caloric tests	VIII, IV, VI, III.
Gag reflex	IX, X.
Tracheal suction	X
Response to pain	Sensory afferents Motor efferents
Apnoea tests	Respiratory centre

Response to pain

Deep pain is produced peripherally by pressure on tender points such as the nail beds and centrally by pressure over the supraorbital nerves, whilst observing for a response from within the cranial nerve distribution. Peripheral non-purposeful movements in response to peripheral pain represent spinal reflexes which are not significant. Simplistically these reflect the loss of descending control over the spinal cord from higher centres. Relatives and attending staff should be warned of these and their significance explained.

Apnoea test

The patient is preoxygenated with 100% O_2, and then disconnected from the ventilator and connected to an anaesthetic breathing circuit with high flow 100% O_2. If the lungs are healthy, oxygenation is maintained by diffusion and the $Paco_2$ rises gradually. The $Paco_2$ must be allowed to rise to a level at which the patient could be expected to breathe. That is a $Paco_2$ of 6.6 kPa for a normal patient but higher in patients with chronic lung disease. If pulmonary function is poor there is a risk of profound hypoxia and cardiac arrest during apnoea testing. In such cases ventilate with added CO_2 or add a deadspace into the circuit, then briefly disconnect the ventilator to look for respiratory movement.

Disconnection of ventilator

When all preconditions are met and two sets of tests confirm brain death the patient is legally dead. The ventilator may be disconnected, and the resulting hypoxia and hypercarbia rapidly results in cardiac standstill. This may be performed soon after tests or later after organ donation if this occurs. The family should be offered the opportunity to sit with the patient and allowed time for distant relatives to visit. At the time of ventilator disconnection they may choose to stay with the patient. Alternatively some prefer to say their farewells before the event and leave or visit later.

ORGAN DONATION

Once brain-stem death has been established the possibility of organ donation arises.

Consent to donation

Theoretically, an organ donor card signed by the patient is all that is required to enable organ donation to take place after the establishment of brain-stem death. The donation of organs, however is crucially dependant on positive public perceptions of the scheme. As a result, in the UK, relatives are almost always asked to give consent, and organs would not be taken in the absence of relatives' consent, even in the presence of a signed donor card. Regrettably in the UK up to half of all relatives will refuse donation (See Ethical & legal issues p. 8.)

 Warning! You must seek the coroner's permission for organ donation from those patients whose death would normally require referral to the coroner. (See Reporting deaths to the coroner p. 15.)

The correct time to approach the subject of organ donation will depend upon the individual circumstances of the case. Relatives will often discuss the subject informally with staff and it is reasonable to explain about the possibility of donation at any time once the possibility of brain-stem death and tests are raised. However, the diagnosis of brain-stem death and the request for organ donation are separate issues. You certainly should not make any formal approach until brain-stem death has been confirmed. Most transplant coordinators are willing to come and speak to relatives about donation if required.

Practicalities of donor management

Transplant surgeons are accepting organs (particularly kidneys) from more unstable and elderly patients than in the past, and in addition there is increasing utilization of tissue such as bone, skin and heart valves. If in doubt about what can be used ask the transplant co-ordinator. Each region has one or more transplant co-ordinators who will liaise between the organ retrieval teams and the referring hospital. They will also provide advice on the management of the donor.

The management of a potential organ donor is no different from that of other ICU patients, in particular those with brain injury. The optimization of physiological parameters, particularly oxygen delivery, and the avoidance of secondary physiological insults to organ systems is similar in both situations.

Problems after brain death includes:

● There are mixed haemodynamic disturbances – with low CO and/or SVR. Oxygen uptake and CO_2 production may be abnormally low. Large volumes of fluid may be required to maintain adequate filling pressures and inotropes/vasopressors are frequently necessary to maintain adequate perfusion pressures. Optimization of haemodynamics may require a PA catheter in unstable cases.

● Poor gas exchange is common (e.g. neurogenic pulmonary oedema), and frequently lungs are unsuitable for transplantation. Ventilation should be optimized.

● Pituitary function is impaired in brain death. There is no proven benefit in terms of donor organ function from the administration of steroids or thyroid hormones. Diabetes insipidus is common, use DDAVP (0.5–1 µg IM, IV) as necessary to reduce urine output to sensible volumes.

● Temperature regulation is lost. Warm IV fluids and inspired gases, and warm air blankets will allow the patient to be maintained at normothermia.

Special investigations

● A number of tests need to be carried out before organ donation. There are increasing concerns in relation to donor transmitted disease and the transplant co-ordinator will give advice, as this is a changing area, particularly in relation to hepatitis serology. Usually all tests are sent to one regional laboratory.

Tests prior to donation
Tissue typing
HIV
Hepatitis screening
U & Es
Glucose
LFTs & amylase.
ECG
CXR
Height & girth measurements

SPINAL CORD INJURY

Spinal cord injury may occur as a result of trauma, bony collapse, infection, tumours, infarcts and other pathologies. In all cases of trauma assume that the neck is injured until proven otherwise and immobilize it as part of initial resuscitation.

 Warning! X-rays of the cervical spine do not exclude instability resulting from ligamentous injury or spinal cord damage which can only be excluded by clinical examination in an awake cooperative patient. Therefore, even if X-rays are normal you should maintain immobilization.

Early management of spinal cord injury

● Immobilize the spine to prevent secondary damage. Cervical collar. Tape head to trolley, and use sandbags. (Log roll with in-line stabilization to control head and neck movement.)

● IV access to support BP. Sympathetic blockade from cord injury will produce hypotension and bradycardia depending upon the level. Patients rarely require inotropes to maintain circulation following isolated spinal injury. Look for haemorrhage from other injures (e.g. 'silent' abdomen.)

● Intubation may be required for respiratory insufficiency, or surgery. Consider awake intubation using local anaesthesia (fibreoptic or conventional). Alternatively intubate the anaesthetized patient with in-line immobilization of the neck. Use of gum elastic bougie and McCoy laryngoscope limits the need to extend the neck. Use of suxamethonium is allowed in first few hours after injury. Avoid after 24 hours because of potential for massive K^+ release. (See suxamethonium, p. 29.)

● Urinary retention is a significant cause of spinal hyper-reflexia. Perform early urinary catheterization.

● Gastric stasis is common, pass nasogastric/orogastric tube.

High-dose steroids (methylprednisolone), if given early, may have beneficial effects in spinal injury. Discuss the management with the local spinal injuries unit or spinal surgeon. The indications for early spinal decompression and surgical stabilization are controversial. Transfer to a spinal injury unit only after exclusion and stabilization of other injuries in a general/neurosurgical unit.

NEUROMUSCULAR CONDITIONS

Neuromuscular conditions are important in intensive care practice. The characteristics of the various conditions vary in detail and many patients will never have a clearcut diagnosis made. However, you should consider all such patients to be at risk from the following:

● Incipient respiratory failure. Commonly follows chest infections or major surgery.

● Bulbar palsy leading to recurrent pulmonary aspiration.

● Autonomic neuropathy leads to cardiovascular instability. Bradycardias, tachycardias, hypertension or hypotension may all occur.

● Cardiomyopathy – there is a risk of arrythmias and sudden death.

● Profound sensitivity to muscle relaxants. There may be long lasting weakness after non-depolarizing drugs. Massive K^+ release after suxamethonium is well recognized even before clinical manifestations are seen (avoid using it!).

In most neumusucular conditions patients will have a normal conscious level. If they are paralysed and ventilator-dependant they may be unable to move or show any sign of distress. (The only means of communication may be by blinking the eyelids!) It should be assumed that they are conscious until proved otherwise.

Patients with neuromuscular conditions require supportive care (assisted ventilation, tracheostomy, non-invasive ventilation, nutrition, physiotherapy, etc.). Increasing numbers of such patients are managed on non-invasive home ventilation. Severe kyphoscoliosis is a significant feature in many patients. Occasionally patients who have difficulty in weaning from assisted ventilation are found to have previously undiagnosed neuromuscular disease. The commoner conditions encountered are discussed below.

Myasthenia gravis

This autoimmune disease results from antibodies to the cholinergic receptors in the neuromuscular junction. The mainstay of treatment is with anticholinesterase drugs which increase the level of acetylcholine available at the cholinergic receptors.

Deterioration, increasing muscle weakness and subsequent respiratory failure may result from intercurrent disease, surgery or overdosage of anticholinesterase drugs (cholinergic crisis). In practice by the time myasthenic patients require intensive care it is often difficult to distinguish cholinergic crisis from other causes of muscle fatigue. The short acting anticholinesterase edrophonium may be given to test whether muscle function can be improved ('tensilon test').

Acute exacerbations are treated by increases in anticholinergic drugs, steroids, and plasma exchange. Azathioprine, cyclophosphamide, and thymectomy are useful treatments in the longer term.

Guillain-Barré syndrome

This condition of ascending muscle paralysis usually follows an intercurrent illness. The early use of intravenous immunoglobulin and plasmapharesis may reduce the need for assisted ventilation. Patients who require assisted ventilation may take weeks or months to recover, and recovery is not always complete. Autonomic disturbances are common.

Tetanus

This is very rare in the UK due to successful immunization programmes. It is, however, a major problem abroad. The toxins produced by the bacteria disrupt normal neuromuscular control and produce severe spasms and autonomic disturbances. The management is supportive with wound debridement, antibiotics, immunization and control of spasms and autonomic problems. Severe cases may require protracted sedation and assisted ventilation.

CRITICAL ILLNESS NEUROMYOPATHY

As more and more critically ill patients survive, increasing numbers of patients are developing residual neuromuscular problems; the so called 'critical illness neuromyopathy'. The exact aetiology is unclear but severe sepsis, prolonged immobility, poor nutritional status, neuromuscular blocking drugs, and elderly medically unfit patients are all considered risk factors. Typically it is first noticed when a critically ill patient is in the recovery phase of illness and is unable to move limbs. It is important to recognize the diagnosis and appreciate that the patient may be completely awake but unable to move. Craniofacial movements are often relatively spared and the patient's only means of communication or reponse may be to blink.

It is important to rule out other causes of weakness like cervical cord problems. Neurological examination usually reveals a flaccid paralysis. EMG indicates a mixed picture of neuropathy and myopathy. Biopsy, although not routine, shows axonal degeneration with preservation of myelin sheaths. The condition usually improves over weeks or months and results in a good recovery.

TRAUMA

RESUSCITATION

Depending upon local policy you may be called to assist in the resuscitation of major trauma victims. You should be familiar with ATLS protocols.

Airway (with cervical spine control)

● Assess the adequacy of the airway. Clear upper airway with suction and simple airway manoeuvres and provide 100% oxygen by reservoir bag.
● If necessary secure the airway by intubation or cricothyrotomy depending on clinical situation and degree of urgency.

 Warning! The cervical spine should be assumed to be unstable and must be protected at all times. Use in-line immobilization; sandbag and tape the head to prevent unnecessary movement.

(See Spinal cord injury p. 185).

Breathing

● Support ventilation if necessary.
● Expose the chest and examine for adequacy of respiration. Identify and treat life threatening conditions such as flail chest, tension pneumothorax, and massive haemothorax.

Circulation

● Stop major haemorrhage by direct pressure.
● Assess the adequacy of circulation. In particular pulse rate, BP, and capillary filling.
● Insert two 14 gauge peripheral intravenous cannulae. If this is not possible then cannulate the femoral vein or consider peripheral venous cut down (e.g. saphenous vein.). In ATLS doctrine CVP lines are used for monitoring and not for resuscitation purposes.
● Send blood for cross-matching.
● Give 2–3 litres of crystalloid. If there is no response continue with colloids and blood products. Fully X-matched blood is preferable but group specific, or non X-matched O negative can be used depending upon circumstances.
● If volume loading does not restore perfusion, consider adrenaline bolus followed by an infusion.

Disability (neurological assessment)

● Assess conscious level, pupil size and obvious neurological deficit. A deteriorating Glasgow coma score, or GCS of 8 or below, is an indication for intubation and ventilation. (See Immediate Management of brain injury, p. 167.)

Exposure and secondary survey

● Once the initial survey is complete and the patient is stabilized be sure that appropriate monitoring is established and investigations have been organised (See Table 10.1).

TABLE 10.1 Investigations and monitoring

Routine Investigations	Monitoring
FBC	ECG
U & Es, glucose	Non-invasive BP
ABGs	Pulse oximeter
(Pregnancy test)	CVP
ECG	Urine output
Lateral C-spine X-ray CXR Pelvic X-ray	
Urine (stick test)	

● Completely expose the patient and systematically examine from head to toe looking for other injuries. Include log roll to examine the back and spine and rectal and vaginal examinations.

● Urinary catheters and nasogastric tubes can be inserted if there are no contraindications.

Following resuscitation, stabilization and re-evaluation of the patient, further management can be planned. This may include additional investigations such as diagnostic peritoneal lavage, CT scan, or immediate surgery for life threatening injuries. Multiply injured patients will frequently be eventually transferred for intensive care.

INTENSIVE CARE MANAGEMENT

Care of the multiply injured patient is essentially no different to care of any other ICU patient. Multiple trauma is by its nature a multiple-system disorder, rather than a collection of isolated injuries. Treatment is generally supportive, with appropriate intervention for problems as they are identified.

The following discussion is limited to common problems of direct relevance to care in ICU. Although details relate to accidental trauma they relate equally well to trauma from surgical procedures, burns or other injury.

Multiple-organ failure after trauma

Multiple-organ failure is common after massive trauma. Typically 24–48 hours after apparently adequate resuscitation MOF will supervene. Patients may develop SIRS. Tissue damage, massive blood transfusion, and activation of the cytokine cascade are all implicated but exact mechanisms are unclear. Treatment is largely supportive once necrotic tissue and infection are excluded. (See Sepsis and SIRS p. 200.)

Outcomes

The outcome following major trauma is critically dependant on the site of trauma. Brain injury greatly increases the risk of disability and death. There is clear relationship between increasing number and severity of injuries and death. Age is an important independent variable. Mortality increases with age and the very elderly often die after apparently minor chest or long bone injury.

A number of scoring systems have been described in trauma. The most important of these is injury severity score (ISS). It is descriptively and prognostically valuable. An ISS of greater than 16 is taken to represent major injuries and has a risk of death at around 10%. (See also Prediction of outcome and APACHE, p. 5 & p. 40.)

SPECIFIC INJURIES

Head injury
(See Brain injury, p. 166.)

Facial

In the unconscious or obtunded patient the airway should be secured early by intubation. With time, swelling may make subsequent reintubation or airway manipulation impossible. Therefore, in severe injuries consideration should be given to early tracheostomy. In the presence of facial or base of skull fractures avoid nasal intubation or nasogastric tubes as these may pass into the cranium. Use the oral route.

Heavy bleeding from facial injuries should not be underestimated. Bleeding from the nose may require nasal packing and use of foley catheters to tamponade bleeding. Seek ENT advice.

Injuries to the jaw often require internal fixation and jaw wiring. Do not be afraid to cut the wires in the event of airway problems. When extubating these patients ensure they are awake and have full return of protective reflexes. Broken teeth may be aspirated. Actively look for them on the CXR, use a lateral film to confirm postion (note position of NG tube to delineate the oesophagus). (See also Airway obstruction, p. 216.)

Cervical spine
(See Spinal cord injury, p. 185.)

Soft tissues in neck

Direct injury to soft tissue of the neck can result in airway compromise due either to haematoma/tissue swelling causing compression of the airway or due to direct injury to the larynx or trachea. Secure the airway by early intubation and seek expert surgical help. Vascular injuries in the neck may compromise cerebral circulation. Bleeding may track down into the chest, resulting in haemothorax or haemomediastinum (very rarely cardiac tamponade).

Chest

Pneumothorax

All trauma related pneumothoraces must be drained. Massive air leaks require bronchoscopy to exclude bronchial rupture. Bronchial rupture should also be suspected in the presence of deceleration injury, mediastinal widening, haemoptysis, first rib or clavicular fractures. An urgent thoracic surgical opinion should be sought, as surgical repair may be appropriate.

Haemothorax

This requires early drainage. Once clot becomes well established it becomes difficult to drain; thoracotomy may then be required. Drainage > 600 ml per hour needs urgent surgical referral. (See Practical Procedures: chest drainage, p. 260.) Ensure good venous access, as decompression of a vascular tear can sometimes occur, resulting in massive haemmorrhage. Use a large drain size, 32 French. Apply low-pressure suction.

Rib fractures

These are significant because of the potential for injury to the underlying viscera. Elderly patients with brittle ribs, may have impressive rib fractures with little underlying injury, whilst children with flexible ribs, may have severe visceral injury without obvious fractures.

- Apical rib fractures are associated with injury to great vessels.
- Mid-zone rib fractures are associated with pulmonary contusions.
- Basal rib fractures are associated with abdominal visceral injury (liver, spleen, kidneys).

Simple rib fractures without major visceral injury can often be managed conservatively. Adequate analgesia (thoracic epidural or patient controlled analgesia, PCA), supplemental oxygen, CPAP, and physiotherapy are useful. In the presence of a significant flail segment and underlying pulmonary contusions IPPV is generally required. Typically ventilation will be required for 7–10 days in such cases. Severe life threatening ARDS may also develop. (See ARDS, p. 98.)

Mediastinal injury

Rapid deceleration injuries can result in injury to the mediastinal contents. In particular traumatic transection of the aorta. Many patients with such injuries will die before reaching hospital but some develop a contained rupture which is at risk of massive rebleeding at any time hours or even days ahead. The typical finding is that of hypertension and widened mediastinum on repeat CXR. Typical features are the following:

- Widened mediastinun.
- Trachea shifted to right by haematoma.
- Oesophagus (look for NG tube) shifted to right.
- Associated fractures 1st and 2nd ribs with underlying pleural blood.

Investigations include aortic angiography and spiral CT scan. Transoesophageal echocardiography may have a role but does not provide all the information required for surgery. Some cases of bleeding into the mediastinum will be venous (which does not require surgery), rather than arterial. Refer the patient to cardiothoracic/vascular surgeons.

Cardiac contusions

Blunt trauma to the myocardium can result in myocardial contusion and even myocardial infarction from damage to the anterior descending coronary artery. A fractured sternum should suggest this diagnosis. Cardiac contusions may result in arrhythmias, and ischaemic injury patterns on ECG. These are often transient and not significant but may require appropriate intervention.

Ruptured diaphragm

Blunt trauma to the abdomen may cause the diaphragm to rupture. This usually occurs on the left due to the protection afforded by the liver on the right. The diagnosis is suggested by abdominal visceral gas shadows in the chest. Confirm by the position of the NG tube or inject X-ray contrast down it. Surgical repair is indicated via the chest or abdomen. Occasional patients have a missed ruptured diaphragm and present later with strangulation of hernia contents. The lesion may be noted incidentally. In this situation do not confuse X-ray appearances with pleural fluid/gas collections needing a chest drain!

Abdomen

Pain, guarding, distension, and presence or absence of bowel sounds cannot be reliably elicited in the unconscious, sedated and ventilated patient. If unrecognized injury or continued intra-abdominal bleeding is suspected seek immediate surgical opinion. Diagnostic peritoneal lavage, plain abdominal films, ultrasound and CT scan may be helpful. If doubt remains laparotomy is appropriate.

Ruptured spleen

Following splenectomy there is greatly increased risk of life threatening infection (particularly pneumococcal). Patients require long-term prophylaxis with penicillin (2 years minimum). Also use immunization with *Pneumococcal, Meningococcal,* and *Haemophilus influenzae* B vaccines. (See local guidelines.)

Ruptured liver

If it is impossible to suture tears adequately, surgeons may pack the liver bed and close the abdomen, with the aim to return to theatre after 48 hours. If haemodynamically stable, patients with liver rupture should be transferred to a specialist unit.

Intra-abdominal bleeding

Intra-abdominal bleeding may result in abdominal tamponade. If intra-abdominal pressure rises above venous pressure then perfusion to the abdominal organs is impaired. The first indication may be a falling urine output. Intra-abdominal pressure can be measured by connecting the urinary catheter to a pressure transducer. The management is surgical exploration. Patients may bleed torrentially when the abdomen is opened. There follows a period of haemodynamic instability following visceral reperfusion. Abdominal distension can also impede diaphragmatic function and make weaning from ventilation difficult.

Pelvis

Pelvic injuries can result in major blood loss. Unstable pelvic injuries are managed by early external fixation which is typically performed in A&E. This helps to reduce bleeding and ultimately allows for earlier mobilization.

Urethral injury should be considered in all cases of pelvic injury. Suspect if there is bleeding from urethral meatus or an abnormal rectal examination. Seek help from urologists. Diagnosis is by a urethrogram (perform in A & E). Management is by suprapubic catheter, with definitive repair at later date.

Limbs

Look for obvious deformity and check for neurovascular integrity. Early reduction of deformity and splinting reduces bleeding and pain.

Compartment syndrome

After initial resuscitation injured areas often become swollen. Swelling of soft tissues in the calf or forearm, where muscles groups are restricted by fascial layers, may result in increased pressure inside the compartments. This restricts blood flow to the muscles which become ischaemic. If left untreated, necrosis and ischaemic contractures may develop. This problem may be seen after fractures, soft tissue damage, prolonged pressure from any cause (e.g. coma), and following vascular surgery.

Causes of compartment syndrome
Forearm fractures
Lower limb fractures
Limb vascular injury/surgery
Crush injury

Look for swollen, tense, and painful muscles (particularly on extension) in the calf and forearm. Pulses may be absent but not invariably so. Compartmental pressure is measured by inserting a 21 gauge (green) needle connected to an intraflow flush device and pressure transducer (as for any intravascular monitoring). Pressures greater than 40 mmHg are an indication for fasciotomy. This can be performed in the ICU. Wounds are left open and closed subsequently when swelling subsides.

Muscle injury

Crush syndrome

This was classically described after lower limb crush injury but can occur following injuries to any muscle group or even from necrotic muscle in surgical wounds. It may follow a missed compartment syndrome. It also occurs following prolonged immobility in drug overdosage, epilepsy or head injury. Muscle breakdown (rhabdomyolysis) releases toxic products into the circulation. These produce a systemic inflammatory response syndrome which may progress to multiple-organ failure. In addition, myoglobin specifically precipitates in renal tubules and causes ARF. The management involves prevention, recognition of the problem and supportive care. Measure creatinine kinase (CK) which is usually greater than 5000 units, and urinary myoglobin (rapidly disappears after a few hours). Exclude and treat compartment syndromes and excise dead muscle (often amputation is required).

Forced alkaline diuresis

Fluid loading and diuretics help maintain urine output. An alkaline diuresis may prevent myoglobin precipitation in the renal tubules. Replace the hourly urine output + 50 ml with alternating hours of 1.4% bicarbonate solution and 5% dextrose. In addition give 0.5 g/kg mannitol. Continue this regimen until resolution of myoglobinuria.

Should renal failure occur, supportive treatment is required. Once renal failure is established the course typically follows that of ATN, with gradual complete recovery of renal function. (See Indications for renal replacement therapy, p. 122.)

Fat embolism

The classic presentation is the onset of dyspnoea, hypoxaemia, petechial rash, and acute confusional state following long bone fracture or orthopaedic instrumentation. The signs are very non-specific and can be caused by pneumonia, sepsis and other complications of trauma and surgery. Fat embolism is often a diagnosis of exclusion.

The mechanisms for this condition are unclear. The simplest explanation is embolization of fat from long bone marrow into the circulation, and then to the lungs and other organs. This does not explain how fat droplets cross the lungs into the systemic circulation to produce CNS effects, nor why most patients do not develop the condition despite the common presence of fat droplets in the circulation after long bone injury.

Investigations

Fat droplets may be seen in retinal vessels, sputum or urine – none of these findings are specific for the condition. CT scan of the brain is usually normal or shows mild diffuse cerebral oedema, MRI scan shows areas of microinfarction.

Management
This is supportive. The usual referral is for respiratory insufficiency which may progress to severe ARDS. The CNS signs usually settle over time but occasional patients develop severe brain injury, with long-term damage or even death.

Although operative intervention may precipitate fat embolism, trauma studies suggest that early orthopaedic fixation of fractures reduces the overall incidence of clinically significant fat embolism.

BURNS

Patients with extensive burns injuries (>20% body surface area) are usually managed in regional burns centres. You may, however, be called to help in the initial resuscitation of a burns victim or may be required to manage the patient in the general ICU because of other coexisting problems.

Resuscitation
The basic principles of resuscitation of the burn victim are the same as for any other patient. The main problems relate to the potential for thermal injuries to the airway, large fluid lossess and potential for infection.

● Give humidified oxygen by face mask. If there are extensive facial burns, or any evidence of thermal injury to the airway, the airway should be secured by endotracheal intubation. This should be performed 'electively' before oedema and swelling make intubation impossible.
● Establish IV access. Where possible avoid siting cannulae through burned skin to reduce the risk of infection.
● Give IV analgesia and commence fluid resuscitation.

The fluid requirements depend on the size of the burn. This is estimated from the rule of nines or from burns charts. A number of regimens are described for fluid replacement based on either crystalloid or colloid infusion. For example:

> 4.5% albumin solution
> 0.5 ml/kg/% burn
> Given over each of six consecutive periods of
> 4, 4, 4, 6, 6, & 12 hours.

It is important to realize that such formulae are a guide only and frequently underestimate fluid requirments. The aim of fluid resuscitation is to restore plasma and extracellular volumes and thus adequate tissue and organ perfusion. Urine output and core–peripheral temperature gradient provide a guide. Many burns units avoid central cannulation because of the risk of infection. However, CVP monitoring and PAC may be required. If there is a clear clinical indication, these are justifiable.

- Monitor electrolytes and haemoglobin/haematocrit.
- Blood may be required to maintain an Hb > 10 g/dl.
- Circumferential burns may require emrgency incision (escharotomy).
- Burns should be covered in sterile drapes or plastic film to reduce infection and fluid loss.
- Major burns cause SIRS. (See Sepsis, p. 200.)

CARBON MONOXIDE POISONING

Carbon monoxide is a product of incomplete combustion. It avidly bonds to haemoglobin, resulting in carboxyhaemoglobin which does not carry oxygen. Severe cases may suffer anoxic brain damage. Carbon monoxide poisoning may be seen in combination with burns, from smoke inhalation, from inadequately ventilated heating appliances (unexplained collapse) and following suicide attempts.

Clinical features of carbon monoxide poisoning

Cherry red colour
Headaches
Nausea & vomiting
Arrhythmias
Seizures
Coma, confusional states

The diagnosis is easily missed. Measure carboxyhaemoglobin levels in all of the situations listed in the box. Levels >20% are significant.

Treatment is supportive. If the inspired oxygen concentration is increased to 100% the half life of carboxyhaemaglobin is 1 hour. Therefore, blood levels will quickly return to normal.

There is evidence, however, that in patients that have had recorded carboxyhaemaglobin levels >20% and/or neurological symptoms at any time, hyperbaric oxygen therapy reduces the incidence of late neurological sequelae.

The benefits of hyperbaric oxygen need to be weighed against the risks of transfer to a specialist centre. Seek advice from poisons centres.

 Warning! Not all UK hyperbaric facilities are based on hospital sites, check before agreeing to go, as you may find yourself in the middle of nowhere!

SEPSIS

SEPSIS SYNDROMES

Sepsis is common in the ICU and accounts for one-quarter of intensive care deaths in the United States. However, the clinical picture seen in overwhelming infection can also be produced by other processes such as the ischaemia reperfusion syndrome, dead tissue, endotoxaemia, liver failure and pancreatitis.

Therefore, in clinical practice sepsis is described as a syndrome rather than a disease process. The following definitions are used.

Systemic inflammatory response syndrome (SIRS)

Disseminated inflammatory response which may be triggered by a wide range of processes. Two or more of the features listed in the box are typical.

Typical features of SIRS

Temperature >38°C or <36°C
Heart rate >90/min
Tachypnoea: a respiratory rate of >20 breaths/min
Hyperventilation: Pa_{CO_2} of <4.3 kPa
An alteration of the WBC count of >12 000 cells/mm³, <4000 cells/mm³, or the presence of >10% immature neutrophils ('bands')

Sepsis

Features of SIRS are present in association with a documented infection. This is typically a Gram-negative bacterium, although Gram-positive organisms, viral, fungal, and protozoal infection may all produce a similar picture.

Severe sepsis and septic shock

Severe sepsis is associated with end organ dysfunction which may include oliguria not responsive to fluid challenge, mental confusion, and the requirement for artificial ventilation. Severe sepsis may be complicated by shock when the systolic blood pressure is <90 mmHg, or 40 mmHg below the patient's habitual blood pressure.

PATHOPHYSIOLOGY

The clinical picture of sepsis (SIRS) may be triggered by a number of factors including infection, tissue ischaemia or the ischaemia – reperfusion syndrome, all of which lead directly or indirectly to activation of the immunoinflammatory cascade described below. There is particular interest, however, in the role of the GI tract in the development of sepsis during critical illness.

In health, the GI mucosa is an effective barrier against enteric organisms and endotoxin. In critical illness, however, inadequate splanchnic perfusion may result in loss of integrity of this barrier allowing bacteria and endotoxin to translocate into the portal circulation. The presence of endotoxin (released from bacteria or translocated from the gut) is a stimulus to the release of tumour necrosis factor (TNFα), platelet activating factor (PAF) and other proinflammatory cytokines. These have many effects including the development of widespread endovascular permeability changes (leakage of fluid from capillaries into the interstitium) vasodilatation (hypotension), sequestration of neutrophils, platelet adhesion, activation of complement and clotting (DIC).

There has been much interest in recent years in manipulation of the cytokine cascade as a means of altering outcome in sepsis. Despite early promise, these attempts have generally proved disappointing. (See also Gastrointestinal tract failure and Gastric tonometery p. 108, 264.)

SEPTIC SHOCK

Clinical features
Patients present with the features of SIRS, hypotension and end organ dysfunction. Additionally there may be a marked metabolic acidosis. Patients are often peripherally shut down and cool. Following fluid resuscitation and in the presence of adequate physiological reserve, circulatory status may be transformed to that of 'warm septic shock'. The circulation becomes hyperdynamic with an elevated cardiac output and reduced systemic vascular resistance. At this stage patients exhibit warm peripheries, flushing and visible cardiac pulsation.

Management
The first imperatives are resuscitation and stabilization. This is followed by investigation of the underlying source of sepsis. The third stage involves management of specific underlying problems and complications.

Resuscitation

● Give oxygen. If end organ failure is compromising respiration (respiratory failure, severe confusion, etc.), early consideration should be given to securing the airway and instituting artificial ventilation.
● Secure venous access.

There is a risk that drugs used to facilitate intubation may cause circulatory decompensation (see Intubation, p. 247), therefore, where ventilation is not required immediately it is often wiser to institute fluid resuscitation and site invasive haemodynamic monitoring (see Arterial cannulation, p. 227), prior to attempting intubation. Peripheral arterial cannulation is not always feasible and in any case may give a poor guide to central arterial pressures. Consider femoral or brachial cannulation.

Small incremental bolus doses of a catecholamine may be necessary at the time of intubation to maintain haemodynamic stability. The drug and dose used will depend on individual circumstances. Consider:

- Adrenaline 1:10 000. Give 0.5 ml (50 µg) increments.
- Phenylepherine 0.01 mg/ml. Give 0.5 ml (5 µg) increments.

Management

Patients with sepsis and septic shock are often grossly hypovolaemic because of vasodilatation and capillary permeability changes leading to third space fluid loss. This situation may well be exacerbated by pyrexia and fluid loss related to any underlying pathology. Vigorous fluid resuscitation may, therefore, be required. There is controversy over whether colloid or crystalloid solutions are more appropriate; on balance it is likely that a combination represents optimal management. Often 2–3 litres of fluid may be required as initial resuscitation volume. Volume loading should be guided by left-sided filling pressures; therefore consider pulmonary artery catheterization at an early stage.

- Give 2–3 litres fluid as initial resuscitation volume (e.g. 2 litres 0.9% saline and 1 litre colloid).
- Establish invasive monitoring. Arterial line if not already in situ and pulmonary artery catheter.
- Optimize volume loading. Initially aim for a PAOP of 15–17 mmHg. Above this level it is unlikely that further fluid loading will produce a further elevation in left ventricular stroke work index. Stroke volume index is often a better guide to filling than left (or right) side atrial pressure; a stroke volume index of 50 ml/m^2 represents a full ventricle.
- Maintain adequate cardiac output (>4.5 l/min/m^2). Consider addition of an inotrope to increase cardiac output (e.g. adrenaline). (See Cardiovascular system p. 49.)
- Maintain adequate tissue perfusion pressure (MAP < 70 mmHg). If MAP remains low despite adequate volume loading and cardiac output, add a vasoconstrictor, e.g. noradrenaline. This should be titrated against BP and not SVR. Patients who maintain an adequate MAP for organ perfusion and urine output despite a low SVR should, therefore, not be commenced on vasopressors; these may reduce tissue oxygen delivery and perfusion.
- Patients with sepsis may be commenced on a low-dose dopaminergic agent (either dopamine at 3 µg/kg/min or dopexamine at 0.5–1 µg/kg/min) to maintain renal and splanchnic perfusion.

Therapeutic end points involve adequate clinical organ and tissue perfusion, e.g. warm pink peripheries, adequate urine output, mentally alert (if not sedated). In addition ensure adequate oxygen delivery. Typically, the oxygen delivery index (DO_2I) should exceed 600 ml/min/m^2. Ensure:

- Adequate oxygen saturation > 94%.
- Adequate haemoglobin, ideally an Hb of 12–13 g/dl should be sought providing there is no contraindication to this. (See Oxygen delivery, p. 40.)

If despite these measures profound hypotension persists, there may be a significant metabolic acidosis (pH < 7.2) or reduced serum ionized calcium (Ca^{2+}_i < 0.8 mmol/l). Consider correction of these metabolic abnormalities as appropriate.

● 50 mmol of 8.4% sodium bicarbonate.
● 10 mmol of calcium chloride.

Once resuscitation and haemodynamic stabilization are complete, consideration can be given to further investigation of underlying causes of sepsis.

Investigation of unexplained sepsis

Any patient who presents with unexplained sepsis in the ICU should have a thorough examination to identify possible causes. Appropriate microbiological samples should be obtained prior to the institution of antibiotic therapy. These should ideally include 'clean stab' blood cultures from a peripheral vein (not from an existing line), sputum or bronchoalveolar lavage for microscopy and culture and urine culture. Bear in mind that existing intensive care patients developing new episodes of sepsis may have line related infections. Consider changing all existing arterial and venous lines and send the tips for culture.

Additional investigations will be guided by the clinical picture and may include those in Table 11.1.

TABLE 11.1 Investigation of unexplained sepsis	
Apparent Source	**Investigation**
Embolic	Culture/change indwelling vascular lines
	Precordial or transoesophageal echo-cardiography
Chest	CXR
	Bronchoscopy + BAL
	Tap & culture pleural fluid
	CT scan
Abdomen & Pelvis	Amylase
	Culture drain fluids (fresh samples)
	Tap & culture ascites
	Abdominal & pelvic ultrasound
	Abdominal & pelvic CT scan
	Laparotomy
Wounds	Pus or tissue (Swabs if nothing else available)
CNS	CT scan
	Lumbar puncture

In practice the largest patient group is those with intra-abdominal sepsis. Abdominal ultrasound and CT scan are likely to be the most valuable investigation. Labelled white cell scanning may rarely be valuable to locate collections of pus. If pus or abscesses are confirmed these should be imaged, drained and cultured. In the absence of an identifiable cause of sepsis, and in the face of a deteriorating clinical picture, laparotomy may be warranted. Seek senior advice and a surgical opinion.

Pyrexia of unknown origin

If the cause of sepsis is not apparent, consider investigation for other causes of pyrexia. Pyrexia of unknown origin may be associated with autoimimmune inflammatory processes (autoantibodies and vasculitic screen), malignancy, drugs and rare infectious diseases. Seek advice.

Complications

The specific complications and pattern of organ dysfunction will vary from patient to patient. A large number of patients will require renal support, some patients may develop prolonged GI tract failure and a large proportion will develop ARDS or coagulopathy. Some patients will develop multiple organ dysfunction. Specific supportive measures for each system should be considered (See relevant sections.)

Prognosis

Overall the mortality from sepsis with shock remains high ranging from 30–70% in various studies. Best results are likely to be obtained by persistence and great attention to detail.

EMPIRICAL ANTIBIOTIC THERAPY

In general, unless patients are at high risk (e.g. immunocompromized), antibiotic therapy is best withheld until a positive microbiological diagnosis is made. In up to 50% of cases of severe sepsis and septic shock, however, no positive microbiological sample is ever obtained and antibiotics may have to be started on an empirical basis. Table 11.2 is a guide only. You should follow your hospital antibiotic policy or ask advice from your hospital microbiologist.

TABLE 11.2 Empirical antibiotic therapy in sepsis

Source	Common pathogens	Suggested antibiotic
Community acquired pneumonia	*Strep. pneumoniae* *Haemophilus influenzae*	Cefuroxime and erythromycin
Including possible atypical pneumonia	*Legionella* *Mycoplasma* *Chlamydia* *Coxiella*	
	If *Staph. aureus* suspected	Add flucloxacillin
	If *Pneumocystis carinii* suspected	High dose co-trimoxazole
Nosocomial pneumonia	*Strep. pneumoniae* *Haemophilus influenzae* Enterobacteria	Cefuroxime
		(If previously treated ciprofloxacin or ceftazidime)
Intraabdominal sepsis	Staphylococci Enterobacteria Anaerobes	Cefuroxime and metronidazole (5–7 days)
		(If previously treated, gentamicin, amoxycillin and metronidazole or ceftazidime and metronidazole)
Pelvic infection	Anaerobes Enterobacteria	Cefuroxime and metronidazole
Urinary tract	*Eschericia coli* *Proteus* species *Klebsiella* species	Cefuroxime
Wound infection	*Staph. aureus** Streptococci Enterobacteria	Amoxycillin, flucloxacillin, (Add metronidazole for traumatic wounds)
Necrotizing fasciitis	Mixed synergystic flora	Benzyl penicillin, gentamicin and metronidazole
	If Group A strep.	Benzyl penicillin ± clindamycin
IV Line sepsis (remove line)	*Staph. aureus** Coag. neg. staph. Streptococci Enterococci Gram-neg. species	Flucloxacillin and ceftazidine
Meningitis	*Neisseria meningitidis* *Strep. pneumoniae* *Haemophilus influenzae*	Cefotaxime

*If MRSA possible: consider vancomycin (see below).

SPECIFIC INFECTIONS ON ICU

GRAM-POSITIVE BACTERIA

Methicillin resistant staphylococcus aureus (MRSA)

Infection due to *Staphylococcus aureus* is common and there is increasingly a problem with MRSA. These strains are resistant to all the standard antibiotics. The only reliable antibiotics against MRSA are vancomycin and teicoplanin. Outbreaks of infection have occured in some ICUs and are difficult to control. Patients are usually isolated in side rooms and scrupulously barrier-nursed. Seek advice from a microbiologist and/or hospital infection control team.

Coagulase-negative staphylococci

Coagulase-negative staphylococci (e.g. *Staph. epidermidis*) are part of the normal skin flora. They have a predilection for sticking to plastic devices and commonly colonize indwelling central venous lines. They may cause systemic infection and are often multiply resistant to antibiotics. If suspected remove or change indwelling lines and discuss with a microbiologist. Genuine infection requires vancomycin or teicoplanin.

Enterococci

Enterococci are part of the normal flora of the GI tract and female genital tract, but in ICU patients they may be responsible for bacteraemia, endocarditis, urinary tract and wound infections. They are usually sensitive to ampicillin or a combination of ampicillin and aminoglycoside but there is increasing incidence of antibiotic resistance. Seek advice.

GRAM-NEGATIVE BACTERIA

Escherichia coli, *Klebsiella* and coliforms

These gram-negative bacteria are normal commensals in the gastrointestinal tract but are a significant cause of infection on the ICU. They typically infect the respiratory tract, urinary tract, and wounds, and may lead to bacteraemia, septicaemia and septic shock. Cephalosporins can be used as first-line treatment, but again there is increasing antibiotic resistance. Seek advice.

Pseudomonas

The overall incidence of *Pseudomonas* infection in ICU seems to be declining. However, it remains a serious problem, particularly affecting the respiratory tract. Antibiotic resistance is widespread, but aminoglycosides, ceftazadime, imipenem, and ciprofloxacin are useful. Seek advice from your microbiologist, who will be aware of local resistance patterns.

Acinetobacter species

These gram-negative coccobacilli are widespread in the environment. They are increasingly recognized as an important pathogen in ICU patients, particularly causing respiratory tract and wound infection and occasionally bacteraemias. They are frequently multiply resistant to antibiotics. Seek advice.

FUNGAL INFECTION

Fungal infection on the ICU is increasingly recognized particularly among patients who are severely compromised and who have received multiple courses of broad-spectrum antibiotics. *Candida albicans* is the most common species. Diagnosis is difficult, but the presence of topical candida infection at more than one site (e.g. oral, genital wounds) should raise suspicion. Fungi grow poorly in conventional blood culture bottles, and serological markers (e.g. *Candida, Aspergillus* antigen tests) may be helpful, although this may not distinguish colonization from infection. Empirical treatment with antifungals may sometimes be appropriate. Seek advice.

MENINGOCOCCAL SEPSIS

Neisseria meningitidis is a gram-negative diplococci which approximately 10% of the population carry as a nasal commensal. It causes a spectrum of illness from meningitis (without systemic sepsis) to a full blown septicaemia illness. (See also Meningitis, p. 181.)

Although meningococcal sepsis is most common in paediatric intensive care occasional cases occur in young adults. It can be a devastating illness resulting in death within a few hours. You should always seek senior help.

Diagnosis

Early symptoms of systemic infection include fever (often > 40°C), arthralgia, myalgia, headache and vomiting. The diagnosis of meningococcal sepsis is made on the basis of the typical purpuric rash together with evidence of hypotension, tachycardia, and poor perfusion.

 Warning! The diagnosis of meningococcal sepsis is based initially on clinical signs. Life saving antibiotic treatment (cefotaxime or benzyl penicillin) and resuscitation should be commenced immediately. This must not be delayed by investigations.

Management

● Antibiotics should be given as soon as the diagnosis is suspected. High-dose IV cefotaxime is a suitable choice in the first instance. When meningocccal disease is confirmed benzyl penicillin can be substituted. This does not irradicate nasal carriage and three doses of rifampicin are also given to abolish this (See Prophylaxis below).

● Give 100% oxygen by face mask. May require intubation and ventilation. Beware of cardiovascular collapse!

● Establish IV access. Give colloid (4.5% albumin) to support the circulation. Large volumes are usually required to maintain BP and improve peripheral circulation.

● Establish invasive arterial blood pressure monitoring, central venous access/pulmonary artery catheterization.

● Commence inotropes as required. Typically adrenaline is first line. Start renal dose dopamine.

● Peripheral and digitial ischemia. If blood pressure is adequate consider prostacycline infusion 5–10 ng/kg/min. This improves microvascular perfusion and may reduce risks of digital ischemia.

● Coagulopathy and DIC is common. Send coagulation screen and give FFP, platelets and cryoprecipitate as necessary.

● Hypocalcaemia is common. Consider calcium bolus and possible calcium infusion.

● Metabolic acidosis is the norm. This will improve as the patient's condition improves. Do not give bicarbonate unless extreme (pH < 7.1) or inotropes ineffective.

● Steroids are not routinely indicated. The significance of adrenal haemorrhage (Fredericks–Waterhouse syndrome) is not clear, but if adrenal insufficiency is suspected then replacement steroid therapy is appropriate.

There is increasing use of haemofiltration and plasma exchange in meningococcal sepsis to remove endotoxin, cytokines and other factors, in an attempt to improve overall survival and also to reduce the incidence of sequelae such as digital ischemia. The benefits of these treatments are as yet not proven. You should seek senior advice.

Prophylaxis

Most cases of meningococcal disease are sporadic and 'outbreaks' of infection are rare. However, the index patient, direct family contacts and other close contacts require prophylactic treatment with rifampicin to abolish nasal carriage of meningococcus. This is organized by the public health department and the case should be reported to them as soon as possible.

It is generally considered that there is no need for medical or nursing staff involved in the care of these patients to receive prophylaxis unless direct contamination has occured.

CHAPTER 12

MISCELLANEOUS PROBLEMS

THE POSTOPERATIVE PERIOD

Patients are frequently admitted to ICU following prolonged or complex surgery for a period of monitoring, ventilation, cardiovascular support and stabilization, prior to discharge to a high dependency area or ward. Admission to the ICU may be planned, due to pre-existing disease and/or the nature of the surgery, or may be unplanned as a result of unexpected difficulties in the perioperative period. These may include the following.

Effects of prolonged surgery

Anaesthesia and surgery may be prolonged because of the extensive nature of the procedure or because of technical complexity. Problems may include hypothermia, atelectasis, dehydration and fluid loss, anaesthetic drug accumulation, and the effects of pressure including the development of compartment syndromes.

Delayed recovery from anaesthesia

Causes of delayed recovery from anaesthesia
Effect of CNS depressant drugs
Premedication
Induction agents
Volatile anaesthetic agents
Opiates
Other centrally acting drugs
Other causes
Hypoxia
Hypercarbia
Hypotension
Hypoglycaemia
Metabolic encephalopathy
Hypothermia
TIA/CVA

The causes of delayed recovery (awakening) following anaesthesia are often multifactorial. It may be impossible initially to determine which is the predominant problem. It usually resolves with a period of supportive care in the ICU with patients gradually recovering over a few hours or days.

Prolonged neuromuscular block

Muscle relaxants are used extensively in anaesthesia to facilitate tracheal intubation, provide relaxation for surgical procedures, and to allow lighter planes of general anaesthesia. In the ICU, patients are usually left to clear muscle relaxants without use of reversal agents. Following anaesthesia, the recovery of neuromuscular function is often hastened by the use of anticholinesterase drugs (e.g. neostigmine). These increase the concentration of acetylcholine at the neuromuscular junction and thus competitively reverse the effects of non-depolarizing neuromuscular blocking drugs. They are used in combination with glycopyrrolate which reduces the undesirable (muscarininc) effects of acetylcholine. Typical doses are:

● Neostigmine 2.5 mg + glycopyrrolate 0.5 mg.

Problems relating to residual paralysis are less common since the introduction of newer shorter acting drugs like atracurium. Occasionally, however, there may be delayed recovery of neuromuscular function. A number of factors may contribute to this.

Factors contributing to delayed recovery neuromuscular blockade
Elderly, frail, medically unfit patients
Relative overdose
Renal or liver dysfunction
Underlying neuromuscular disease
Effects of other drugs (e.g. aminoglycosides)
Electrolyte abnormalities
Hypothermia

Patients exhibit jerky movements, make poor respiratory effort and have marked fade on train of four. (See Muscle relaxants p. 28.)

● Give oxygen. Support ventilation if necessary.
● If the patient has some neuromuscular function it may be appropriate to administer a second dose of reversal agent and reassess the situation.
● If this fails to improve the situation or if the patient has minimal neuromuscular function the patient should be resedated, intubated and ventilated until return of neuromuscular function. Remember to explain to the patient what is happening. They may be paralysed but aware of their surroundings.

Hereditary cholinesterase deficiency (1:3000 population) is a specific cause of delayed recovery of neuromuscular function resulting from the delayed metabolism of suxamethonium (and mivacurium). Muscle function usually returns in 2–6 hours. FFP repletes cholinesterase and speeds return of motor power, but is not usually necessary. Send blood to regional centre for identification of particular pattern of cholinesterase deficiency. (See Suxamethonium p. 29.)

Respiratory insufficiency

Postoperative respiratory insufficiency may be predictable in patients with pre-existing respiratory disease and this may be an indication for elective postoperative ventilation. In other patients respiratory insufficiency may arise for a number of reasons and the problem is often multifactorial.

Causes of postoperative respiratory insufficiency

Residual effects of anaesthetic drugs
Residual effects of neuromuscular blockade
Airway obstruction
Bronchospasm
Pre-existing respiratory disease
Pulmonary collapse/consolidation/ARDS
Pneumothorax
Pulmonary oedema
Cardiovascular instability
Sepsis
Hypothermia

Many of these problems are resolved by a short period of ventilation in the ICU combined with simple measures. (See also Respiratory failure p. 78.)

Cardiovascular instability

Cardiovascular instability may arise due to pre-existing cardiovascular disease, from the predictable effects of the surgery, particularly when large fluid losses are expected, or as a result of untoward cardiovascular events.

Causes of postoperative CVS instability

Pre-existing CVS disease.
Myocardial ischaemia/infarction
Fluid losses & bleeding
Fluid overload.
Effects of drugs
Effects of epidural/spinal anaesthesia.
Sepsis
Hypothermia

Many of these problems are solved by simple attention to details of fluid balance as the patient warms up after surgery. More difficult cases may require full invasive monitoring and cardiovascular support. (See Optimizing haemodynamic status, p. 49.)

ICU MANAGEMENT OF THE POSTOPERATIVE PATIENT

The postoperative admission to intensive care of patients allows for:

● Controlled recovery from effects of anaesthesia and surgery.
● Period of rewarming.
● Optimization of respiratory function and controlled weaning from ventilation.
● Optimization of cardiovascular function.
● Monitoring of other organ function, e.g. renal output.
● Adequate analgesia.

When an elective postoperative patient is admitted to the ICU you should be sure that the management plan is agreed with the referring anaesthetist and surgeon. A typical approach is given below:

● Continue ventilation.
● Maintain sedation and analgesia by infusion using short acting drugs such as propofol and alfentanil. Muscle relaxants are generally discontinued unless there is an indication to continue them.
● Assess the patient fully and decide on priorities for management. Send blood for FBC, clotting screen, U&Es and arterial blood gases. Correct abnormalities as necessary.
● Rewarm patient using warm air blanket if necessary. As temperature increases the peripheral circulation will open up (reduction in core–peripheral temperature gradient). Give fluid (colloid or blood) as necessary to maintain adequate circulating volume.
● Metabolic acidosis usually improves as the patient rewarms and circulation improves. Any inotropes can be gradually reduced.

The aim is to achieve a warm, cardiovascular stable patient, requiring minimal inotropic support, with minimal fluid/blood requirements, adequate urine output and satisfactory arterial blood gases. Depending on the premorbid condition of the patient and the nature of the surgery, this can often be achieved after a few hours (e.g. overnight). The sedation can then be reduced and the patient woken up and extubated as appropriate.

Aortic aneurysm repair

Following elective aortic aneurysm repair patients can generally be allowed to warm up and extubate after a few hours as described above. Emergency aneurysm repairs may be more unstable and the management will depend upon individual circumstances. Control of BP is important. This should be maintained at a level which is normal for the patient to ensure adequate perfusion of vital organs, in particular the kidneys. At the same time significant hypertension should be avoided in order to prevent undue strain on the vascular anastomosis. This may require use of nifedipine or GTN infusion, especially during the phase of emergence from sedation.

Persistent ischaemia of the lower limbs despite optimization of haemodynamic status, may require embolectomy or exploration of the graft. Seek surgical opinion. (See Hypertension, p. 56.)

Free tissue transfer (free flap)

The management of patients following free tissue transfer is similar to that described above. In addition, however, the adequate perfusion and survival of the graft is paramount.

The normal mechanisms controlling blood flow in the grafted tissue are destroyed. The circulation to the graft is essentially passive and depends entirely on the flow through the feeding vessels. Therefore, colloid should be used to maintain the patient's circulation as full as possible, as measured by CVP, urine output and core–peripheral temperature gradient. The response to any deterioration in these parameters should be to give further fluid. At the same time the denervated vessels of the graft are highly sensitive to circulating catecholamines (endogenous or exogenous). Adequate analgesia is, therefore, essential. The patient should be kept as warm as possible and inotropes/vasoconstricting drugs should be avoided except in extremis. Dopexamine may be of value in improving graft blood flow and survival. Seek advice.

If despite these measures graft perfusion appears impaired (dusky/congested/swollen) call the surgical team immediately. The vascular pedicles and anastomosis may need surgical exploration.

Transplants

Transplants are a special form of free tissue transfer. The principles are similar to those described above with particular management issues depending on the particular organ involved. These procedures are only carried out in specialist centres and you should seek senior advice.

POSTOPERATIVE ANALGESIA

Patient controlled analgesia (PCAs)

These techniques are extensively used to provide analgesia particularly in postoperative patients. Typically the patient will be established on such a device prior to transfer to a general ward. Although not intended for operation by nurses they may be used safely and conveniently in this way in an ICU setting.

Care should be taken in setting devices up, a dedicated line or non-return valve should be used. There have been a number of problems due to excessive background dosing, surges of morphine on unblocking IV lines, and siphoning of contents out of syringes. Avoid background infusions if possible. Put syringe drivers below level of patient. (For typical regimes see Sedation and analgesia, p. 24.)

Regional blockade

An increasing number of patients undergoing major surgery have analgesia provided by the epidural and spinal route. These techniques may also be used to relieve pain from trauma (e.g. fractured ribs) and ischaemic limbs.

Potential advantages include the avoidance of centrally acting sedative analgesic drugs. This results in awake, co-operative and pain-free patients, better able to cough and clear airway secretions. In addition in patients with ischaemic limbs, neuroaxial blockade (which includes sympathetic blockade) may provide both analgesia and improvement in perfusion of the ischaemic limb.

Detailed description of epidural techniques are beyond the scope of this book. When a patient is admitted with an epidural in situ you should make sure that you confirm the analgesic regime with the responsible anaesthetist. Local anaesthetic and opiate drugs may be used alone or in combination. Typical regimes are:

- Bupivacaine 0.01–0.25% by infusion at 5–10 ml/h.
- ± Fentanyl 4 μg/ml.

If break-through pain occurs and the patient is otherwise stable give a 5–8 ml bolus of the epidural solution (or 0.25% plain bupivicaine) and then increase the infusion rate. This is normally effective within 10–15 minutes. Beware of hypotension.

 Warning! Great care must be taken to avoid injection of the wrong drugs or wrong doses into epidural catheters. If you are not familiar with epidural techniques seek help.

Complications of epidural blockade (→ Table 12.1)

TABLE 12.1 Complications of epidural blockade

Local anaesthetics	Opiates
Potential local anaesthetic toxicity	Itching
Hypotension (sympathetic blockade)	CNS depression including apnoea
Muscle weakness (including respiration)	Urinary retention
Bradycardias (block > T4 level)	Nausea and vomiting
Urine retention	
Complete spinal	

- Hypotension usually responds to fluid loading (500 ml colloid) and reducing the rate of epidural infusion. If significant hypotension develops, stop infusion and consider use of vasopressors (e.g. phenylephrine 5 μg increments).
- Muscle weakness is often unavoidable. If block is too high (e.g. involving arms) then reduce the rate of infusion and/or reduce the concentration of local anaesthetic. If respiratory muscle weakness occurs ventilation may be necessary until the effects of the local anaesthetic wear off.
- At the doses used, the addition of opiates to epidural infusion may significantly improve analgesia without significant increase in the side-effect profile. Nausea and itching may be helped by low-dose naloxone without loss of analgesia. CNS depression may require ventilation.

AIRWAY OBSTRUCTION

Airway obstruction is common in the immediate postoperative period while patients are in the recovery room and the effects of anaesthetic drugs wear off. Occasionally airway obstruction may persist or may be a potential risk following a particular surgical procedure. These patients will frequently be admitted to the ICU.

Causes of airway obstruction

Facial trauma
Soft tissue obstruction in upper airway
Bleeding/swelling/tumour/foreign body in upper airway
Vocal cord paralysis following damage to laryngeal nerve/hypocalcaemia
Bleeding/swelling/tumour/foreign body in lower airway
External compression of trachea, e.g. from bleeding/swelling in the neck
Collapse of trachea, e.g. tracheomalacia

It is vital to recognize actual or impending airway obstruction before the patient suffers a hypoxic episode. In the spontaneously breathing patient airway obstruction produces obvious respiratory distress. Tracheal tug, intercostal recession (mostly in children) and paradoxical respiratory movements all indicate significant obstruction. Stridor is typical, but indicates at least some air flow; the silent patient may be in much greater danger.

Management

The management of any patient with airway obstruction is essentially the same, i.e. secure the airway by endotracheal intubation or tracheostomy as soon and as safely as possible. There are, however, a few points to bear in mind depending on the situation and your own experience.

● Do not leave the patient unattended. Do not delay management of the problem by sending the patient for investigations.
● Give oxygen by face mask. Support ventilation with a bag and mask if necessary and practicable.
● Simple manoeuvres such as extending the neck, jaw thrust and suctioning of the airway may improve the situation.
● Seek help from senior anaesthetist and ENT surgeon as appropriate. In these circumstances intubation/reintubation can often be difficult.

The definitive management is to secure the airway by tracheal intubation or tracheostomy. If time allows this should be performed in theatre with surgeons scrubbed and prepared for emergency tracheostomy. Awake fibreoptic intubation, awake tracheostomy or gaseous anaesthetic induction with the patient breathing spontaneously may be appropriate depending on the circumstances. It is beyond the scope of this text to cover these in detail. The usual problem at intubation is gross swelling and distortion of the tissues which mean the laryngeal inlet cannot be visualized. Often the endotracheal tube has to be passed blindly through swollen tissues into the larynx.

Once the airway is secured the management is that of the underlying condition. Allow time for swelling to subside. Steroids may be of value. Elevate the head of the bed, and reassess after 24 hours.

Postoperative bleeding/trauma in the neck

Following surgical procedures in the neck (e.g. thyroidectomy) postoperative bleeding into the tissues of the neck may occasionally produce airway obstruction by direct compression. In an emergency, you should open the surgical wound and decompress the bleeding to relieve pressure on the airway. The wound can then be formally explored by a surgeon in order to achieve haemostasis. If this fails to relieve the problem you should intubate the patient as described above.

Jaw wiring

Patients with fractured mandibles frequently have their jaws wired together to ensure correct dental occlusion whilst the fracture heals. These patients should only be extubated once full consciousness and respiratory effort has returned. They are often admitted to intensive care immediately for observation and monitoring. If airway obstruction occurs (e.g. due to vomiting), you should cut the wires to gain access to the airway and manage the situation as appropriate.

Airway obstruction in the intubated patient

This is common in the ICU and may be due to kinking of the endotracheal tube or the effects of thick secretions, blood clot or even occasionally foreign body. Adequate humidification, regular suctioning and careful fixation of endotracheal tubes, avoids most problems, but these may still arise particularly in children where the endotracheal tube is smaller in diameter and blocks more easily.

It is important to recognize and act on these problems immediately. Typical clues are increased airway pressure, inability to inflate chest manually with a bag, falling SaO_2 and absent $ETCO_2$ trace.

● Ventilate with 100% oxygen if possible. If not remove the endotracheal tube and manually ventilate the patient with a bag and mask before reintubating.

 Warning! Obstruction of the endotracheal tube may not be immediately recognized. If ever in doubt about endotracheal/ tracheosotmy tube patency change the tube.

● If able to ventilate satisfactorily suck out endotracheal tube. Use 10–20 ml saline instilled down endotracheal tube to loosen secretion.
● Bronchoscopy may be helpful.

● In 'ball valve' obstruction the chest can be inflated but exhaled gas is trapped by a plug impinging on the end of the tracheal tube. Apply suction directly to the endotracheal tube and remove it, dragging the plug out at the same time. Ventilate the patient by bag and mask before reintubating.

Postextubation stridor

Airway obstruction and stridor may occur following extubation. This may be as a result of underlying pathology but frequently results from laryngeal oedema, particularly in children whose airways are narrower. This may occasionally require reintubation. Consider dexamethasone.

ANAPHYLACTOID REACTIONS

Anaphylactoid is a term which encompasses all life threatening acute 'allergic' reactions regardless of their exact pathogenesis. It includes true immune mediated type 1 or anaphylactic hypersensitivity reactions. These reactions are relatively uncommon but can result in catastrophic collapse. Causes include drugs, fluids, blood products, latex, nuts and bee stings.

Clinical manifestations

The onset of symptoms may occur within 1–2 minutes of exposure to the precipitating agent or may be delayed up to 1–2 hours and may be modified by the effects of general or regional anaesthesia. The clinical manifestations include:

● Cutaneous flushing urticaria, angioedema.
● Laryngeal oedema, bronchospasm, increased airway pressure.
● Falling SaO_2.
● Tachycardia, hypotension, cardiac arrest.
● Abdominal pain, nausea, vomiting, diarrhoea.

Life-saving treatment depends on early recognition and appropriate management.

Differential diagnosis of anaphylactoid reactions
Vasovagal reaction
Dysrhythmia
Myocardial infarction
Effects of drugs (including illicit drugs)
Pulmonary embolism
Bronchospasm
Pulmonary oedema
Aspiration
Hereditary angioneurotic oedema
Idiopathic urticaria
Serum sickness
Carcinoid tumours

Management

 Warning! A spectrum of reactions exists between mild hypotension with bronchospasm, and full blown collapse and cardiac arrest. Response must be measured against the condition of the patient.

● Stop precipitating drugs.
● Give oxygen. Secure airway by endotracheal intubation as soon as possible. Ventilate and commence external cardiac massage if necessary.
● Establish IV access if not already, and give rapid fluid load, e.g. 2–4 l crystalloid or colloid (remember that synthetic colloids may be the cause of the reaction!).
● Give adrenaline titrated against response.
    — 50–100 µg bolus IV for moderate hypotension
    — 0.5–1.0 mg bolus IV for profound collapse followed by
    — 1–5 µg/min infusion.
● If persistent hypotension consider noradrenaline infusion.
● Establish central venous, pulmonary artery and arterial cathaterization when appropriate. Take blood (EDTA & serum) for later analysis. Measure arterial blood gases. If significant acidosis consider 50–100 mmol sodium bicarbonate. (See Metabolic acidosis, p. 137)
● If persistent bronchospasm consider:
    — nebulized salbutamol 2.5–5 mg
    — aminophylline 5 mg/kg IV (loading dose) followed by 0.5 mg/kg/h.
● Glucocorticoids may reduce late sequelae. Consider:
    — hydrocortisone 200 mg followed by 50 mg 6 hourly
    — methylprednisolone 1 mg/kg initially repeated every 6 hours.
● Antihistamines are of no proven benefit.
● Following resuscitation these patients should be managed in the ICU.
Late reactions can result in clinical deterioration even some hours after initial stabilization.

Evaluation of cause of anaphylactoid reaction

Following anaphylactoid reaction it is important to try and establish the cause so that future reactions may be avoided. Take a detailed history of this and other previous allergic reactions. Blood samples taken as soon after the reaction as possible and at regular intervals thereafter can be analysed for immune markers including antibodies (IGE), complement and mediator levels. These may help elucidate the nature of the reaction rather than the causative agent. Radioallergosorbant Tests (RAST) and interval skin-prick testing may determine the causative agent but this is often inconclusive.

● Seek advice from laboratory services/immunology department.

It is essential that patients and their relatives are made aware of the reaction. In the case of nut allergy or bee-sting anaphylaxis patients are now given prefilled adrenaline injectors for emergency use.

MALIGNANT HYPERPYREXIA (MH)

This is a rare inherited condition in which there is an abnormality of ionic calcium transport in muscles. Following exposure to trigger agents (including volatile anaesthetic agents, suxamethonium) susceptible individuals may develop increased muscle tone, increased metabolic rate and hyperpyrexia.

Features of MH

Increased muscle tone
Increased metabolic rate
Hyperthermia (typically increase >2°C/h)
Rising ETCO$_2$
Falling Sa$_{O_2}$
Mixed respiratory/metabolic acidosis
Hyperkalaemia/hypocalcaemia
Myoglobinuria & renal failure
Cardiac failure/dysrhythmia/cardiac arrest

Management

● Discontinue trigger agents. Monitor ECG, Sa$_{O_2}$, core temperature.
● Intubate if not already. Ventilate with 100%. Monitor ETCO$_2$. Manage hypercarbia by hyperventilation.
● Institute active cooling measures.
● Give dantrolene:
  — 1 mg/kg IV over 10 min repeat as necessary up to 10/mg/kg.
● Monitor blood gases, potassium, and calcium. Treat metabolic acidosis, hyperkalaemia and hypocalcaemia as appropriate.
● Measure urine output and myoglobin. Give fluids and consider dopamine to maintain urine output. Mannitol and sodium bicarbonate increase the clearance of myoglobin (note: dantrolene also contains mannitol to improve clearance of myoglobin).

Following stabilization these patients must be monitored in the ICU. The half life of dantrolene is approximately 5 hours. Occasionally hyperpyrexia may recur, requiring further dantrolene. (See Hyperthermia, p. 145.)

THE OBSTETRIC PATIENT

Any medical condition can present in pregnancy and a small number of obstetric patients are admitted to the ICU each year. The physiological changes associated with pregnancy and the safety of the fetus in utero are important considerations but overall the management is usually the same as in the non-pregnant female.

> **Warning!** All pregnant patients with a large uterus (greater than 20 weeks) must be nursed in the lateral position or with lateral tilt to avoid hypotension and uterine hypoperfusion due to inferior vena caval obstruction.

In addition there are some conditions which may present late in pregnancy that require admission to ICU. In most cases patients will be admitted postdelivery as the primary management of most specific obstetric problems is urgent delivery of the fetoplacental unit.

Pre-eclampsia/eclampsia

Pre-eclampsia is a condition characterized by proteinuria, oedema, and hypertension. Eclampsia which may be preceded, by pre-eclampsia or present acutely, is a more severe manifestation of the same disorder in which there are seizures. These conditions usually occur in late pregnancy but may occasionally present immediately postdelivery. The exact pathogenesis of the condition is not known but urgent delivery of the fetal-placental unit, usually by caesarean section, initiates resolution. However, hypertension and seizures may continue for 48 hours.

> **Warning!** These patients are frequently admitted to ICU for a period of stabilization and support. They are young sick patients, and the management issues are often complex. You should always seek advice. The following notes give some guidance.

● Give oxygen by face mask. Intubate and ventilate if necessary. Beware of rises in blood pressure and intracranial pressure on laryngoscopy/intubation. Bolus alfentanil 10 µg/kg may modify this. Subsequently ensure adequate sedation.
● Control hypertension. Hypertension results from vasoconstriction and is accompanied by reduced plasma volume. Vasodilatation and restoration of plasma volume should proceed synchronously. Use labetalol/nifedipine/hydralazine to control blood pressure. (See Hypertension p. 56.)

● Give colloid fluid challenges to expand plasma volume, and support renal output. Invasive monitoring (CVP & pulmonary artery catheter) may be appropriate.

● Control seizures. Simple measures include benzodiazepines. Consider prophylactic anticonvulsant therapy with phenytoin or magnesium. Magnesium sulphate 4 g (16 mmol) over 20 min followed by infusion magnesium sulphate 1 g (4 mmol) every hour. Monitor magnesium levels, aim for 2.5–3.0 mmol/l.

Complications include disseminated intravascular coagulation (DIC), HELLP syndrome, pulmonary oedema, cerebral oedema, cerebral haemorrhage and renal failure. These should be managed as necessary.

HELLP syndrome

HELLP syndrome (haemolysis, elevated liver enzymes, low platelets) is a distinct condition occurring in the peripartum period but frequently accompanies pre-eclampsia/eclampsia. There are abnormalities of the microvascular circulation associated with red cell destruction and increased platelet consumption. The liver is particularly affected, resulting in some cases in hepatic necrosis and rupture. The clinical features are primarily those of abdominal (right upper quadrant) pain and mild jaundice. Thrombocytopenia may result in bleeding.

TABLE 12.2 Diagnostic criteria	
Haemolysis	Abnormal blood film Hyperbilirubinaemia
Elevated liver enzymes	LDH > 600 U/l AST > 70 U/l
Low platelets	<100 × 10⁹/l

Management is largely supportive. Adequate resuscitation, volume loading and prostacycline infusion may improve microvascular circulation. Platelets are generally unnecessary unless there is active bleeding. Plasma exchange may be of value in severe cases. Seek advice.

Amniotic fluid embolism

This is a rare cause of collapse in obstetric patients but is frequently fatal when it does occur. The presence of amniotic fluid and debris in the maternal circulation produces pulmonary hypertension, hypoxaemia, heart failure and SIRS. There is usually an associated coagulopathy. Management is supportive.

Heart failure

Pregnancy and delivery are characterized by increased physiological demands on the heart. In patients with pre-existing heart disease or pregnancy-related cardiomyopathy the heart may be unable to meet these demands and heart failure supervenes. Management is supportive as for other causes of heart failure. Pregnancy-related cardiomyopathy usually improves after delivery. (See Cardiac failure, p. 69.)

PRACTICAL PROCEDURES

GENERAL INFORMATION

Patients in intensive care require large numbers of practical procedures. The information in this chapter is only intended as a guide. The advice is generalized; you should always read the instructions provided with the equipment that you use, and follow your local hospital guidelines.

 Warning! Always seek senior help if you are not familiar with a procedure.

Consent

Formal consent from the patient or relatives may be appropriate for some procedures, such as tracheostomy, whilst consent may be implied for minor or life saving procedures. In any event, always explain to the even apparently unconscious patients what you intend to do. (See Consent to treatment, p. 9.)

Local anaesthetic

Paralysed and sedated patients in ICU may still feel pain from invasive procedures. Use local anaesthetic for all painful procedures.

Universal precautions

Contamination with blood imposes significant risk to staff from blood-borne infection, particularly hepatitis and HIV infections. Universal precautions should be adopted for all invasive procedures. This should include use of gown, gloves, goggles and face mask (See below).

Universal infection control precautions

These precautions have been developed to prevent the spread of infection; to protect you, your patients and colleagues. It is not always possible to know who has an infection; universal infection control precautions apply to everybody. It is your responsibility to follow these as a basis for good practice.

- Wash your hands thoroughly.
- Cuts or grazes on the hands or forearms should be covered with a waterproof dressing whilst at work. Seek medical advice about any septic or weeping areas.
- Single-use gloves should be worn for direct contact with blood or body fluid, broken skin or mucous membranes. Plastic aprons should be worn if splashing of clothing is likely, and face protection should be worn if there is a risk of blood or body fluid splashing the face.
- Place all sharps directly into a sharps bin; do not manually resheath or break needles. Do not overfill sharps bins, and ensure that the bin is securely fastened before disposal. If you do accidentally cut, scrape or puncture your skin, follow the 'Accidental Inocculation Procedure,' i.e.

  – encourage bleeding, wash with warm soapy water, dry and cover with a
    waterproof dressing
  – report the incident to the senior person in charge and ensure a report is
    completed
  – seek advice from the occupational health department or from A & E medicine.
● Clinical waste should be discarded into colour coded bags for incineration.
● Blood or body fluid spills should be disinfected immediately; follow instructions.

   Always follow guidelines and safety information that apply to your
department. If you need further information talk in the first place to a senior
member of staff. Where necessary, further advice can be obtained from specialists
in microbiology, infection control, occupational health, COSHH, health & safety, etc.

Aseptic technique

ICU patients are generally severely debilitated and at risk of infection.
Therefore, when performing procedures, no matter how minor, good
infection control procedures are important. For all invasive procedures strict
aseptic technique is required.

● Collect all necessary equipment before starting.
● Ensure assistance is available to open packs, etc.
● Wash hands with disinfectant (generally chlorhexidine or iodine).
● Dry hands on towel provided in gown pack.
● Put on gown.
● Put on gloves using closed technique.
● Prepare the equipment on the trolley.
● Prepare the patient by washing with spirit or iodine.
● Place sterile towels around the proposed site to make a sterile field.
● Remember to keep hands up to avoid contamination.

**Warning! It is the responsibility of the person performing a procedure
to dispose of all sharps safely and correctly at the end of the procedure.
Remember: never resheath needles. Deposit needles and other sharps
directly in the burn bin. Do not expect the nurses to clear up after you.
Maintain good relations, clear up your own mess.**

ARTERIAL CANNULATION

Arterial cannulation is one of the most commonly performed procedures in
the ICU. There is, however, an associated risk of morbidity and the indication
for arterial cannulation in the individual patient should be considered
carefully.

Indications

● Haemodynamic monitoring: particularly in situations where non-invasive measurements are inadequate, e.g. where changes in arterial blood pressure are likely to be sudden or profound, at extremes of blood pressure and in the presence of arrhythmias.
● Repeated blood sampling. Especially for repeated arterial blood gas sampling. The complications associated with arterial cannulation are outweighed by the morbidity and inconvenience of repeated arterial puncture.

Contraindications

These are relative. Exercise caution in arteriopaths and do not recannulate an artery where previous vascular compromise has occurred. Where possible avoid areas of local sepsis and trauma, limbs with dialysis fistulae and end arteries such as the brachial artery.

You will need:

● Universal precautions. Sterile gloves.
● Minor dressing pack.
● Skin disinfectant.
● Syringe of local anaesthetic/needle.
● Syringe of heparinized saline flush.
● Arterial cannula (usually 20 G or 22 G).
● Extension line and three-way tap.
● Suture.
● Dressing.

Procedure

Decide which artery to cannulate. The radial artery of the non-dominant hand is preferred. Alternatives include the ulnar, dorsalis pedis and posterior tibial arteries. It is pointless, however, to persist with attempts at peripheral arterial cannulation in patients who are hypotensive and 'shut down'. The femoral and brachial arteries are useful during resuscitation of profoundly shocked patients.

Warning! Allen's test: This may be used to establish the adequacy of ulnar collateral circulation to the hand before cannulation of the radial artery. The test is, however, of no proven value. If there is any evidence of vascular compromise the arterial line should be removed and surgical exploration of the artery considered where perfusion is not rapidly restored.

- Arterial cannulation often results in blood spillage. Universal precautions should be used.
- Clean the puncture site and establish a sterile field.
- Gently palpate the artery and inject local anaesthetic to raise a small intradermal bleb at the puncture site 1-cm distal to the proposed cannulation site. Make a small nick in the skin with a 21 G needle.

Either:

- Advance cannula and needle through the puncture site towards the artery at a shallow angle. As the vessel is punctured a flashback of arterial blood is seen in the hub. Holding the needle still, advance the cannula over the needle into the artery. This should be a single smooth movement without resistance.

Or:

- Advance the cannula at a steeper angle and after observing the flashback continue through the artery in order to transfix it. Withdraw the needle slightly from the cannula and then pull the cannula back gently until the tip is in the artery and flashback is observed. Advance cannula into artery.
- Attach extension tubing and three-way tap.
- Aspirate blood from the line to confirm placement and to remove any air bubbles, then flush line with heparinized saline.
- Secure in place by stitching and cover with occlusive dressing. (Do not place stitches to deeply. It is possible to inadvertently tie off peripheral arteries.)
- Attach the arterial line to a pressure transducer and flushing device.

An alternative method for arterial cannulation utilizes a Seldinger technique. The artery is punctured with a needle through which a guide wire is inserted. The needle is withdrawn and the cannula passed over the guide wire. The guide wire is then discarded. This technique may be more successful for difficult cannulations.

Sampling from arterial lines

- Clean sample port with alcohol swab and attach syringe.
- Aspirate 1–2 ml blood into the syringe and then discard this syringe.
- Aspirate sample into fresh syringe or vacuum container.
- Samples for blood gases should be drawn into preheparinized syringes to prevent damage to the blood gas analyser. Any air in the syringe should be expelled. If not analysed immediately in the ITU, the syringe should be capped and placed on ice.
- Flush the line with heparinized saline and place a clean cap on the sampling port.

Complications of arterial cannulation (Table 13.1)

TABLE 7.1 Causes of hyponatraemia

Immediate	Early	Late
Bleeding	Arterial embolism	Infection
Haematoma	Vasospasm	Ulceration
Arterial damage		Thrombosis
		Arteriovenous fistulae

Vascular compromise may occur at any stage. Inadvertent injection of drugs into an arterial line is an important avoidable cause of morbidity and all lines should be clearly labelled. Risk of infection increases with time. Any manifestly infected line should be removed, otherwise lines should be changed regularly according to local protocol (typically every 4–7 days).

After removing arterial lines press firmly for at least 5 minutes. Occasionally persistent bleeding may require a suture (5/0 nylon), to close the skin wound and then further pressure.

PRESSURE TRANSDUCERS

A transducer converts one type of energy (e.g. arterial pressure) into another (e.g. electrical impulse). There are a number of different types of transducer available but the principle is similar for all.

● The patient's arterial line is connected to the transducer by a continuous column of heparinized saline. A pressurized flushing device maintains a small forward flow (approx. 2–3 ml/h) to keep the cannula patent.
● Pressure changes in the vessel are transmitted via the saline to a diaphragm. As this diaphragm moves in response to the pressure changes, its electrical conductivity changes. This results in fluctuations in electrical signal from the diaphragm which is interpreted by a monitor and displayed as an arterial wave form and blood pressure value.

Using transducers

In order for the arterial wave form and blood pressure recording to be accurate the transducer must be used appropriately. Therefore:

● There must be no air bubble in the connection tubing or transducer chamber. This will damp the trace and produce lower blood pressure values. Flush well before connecting transducer to patient.
● The transducer should be maintained at the level of the left atrium and appropriately zeroed. (If raised above this level the recorded pressure will be too low, and vice versa.)

Zeroing transducers

● To zero transducer turn the three-way tap so transducer is open to air and patient connection is switched off. The transducer is now connected to atmospheric or zero gauge pressure.
● Zero the monitoring system as per manufacturer's instructions. (There is usually a single button to press.)
● When zeroing complete, turn three-way tap back to reconnect patient to the transducer. Check that the trace and values obtained are as expected.

COMMON PROBLEM: INVASIVE AND NON-INVASIVE PRESSURE MONITORING DISAGREE

Occasionally the blood pressure displayed by the invasive arterial monitoring differs from that obtained by non-invasive methods (i.e. blood pressure cuff). This is generally because of either excessive damping or resonance in the invasive monitoring in which case the mean arterial pressures are usually in close agreement.

● Check the arterial line is correctly sited and flush lumen with heparinized saline.
● Check that there are no air bubbles in the connecting tubing or transducer chamber.
● Check zero on invasive monitoring.

   In some cases, peripheral vasospasm may be a cause of this error. If in doubt, resite the arterial line, or use the non-invasive measurements of blood pressure. In this case, the line can still be retained for arterial blood gas sampling.

CENTRAL VENOUS CANNULATION

Warning! You should not attempt central venous cannulation without supervision until you have been adequately taught to do so. You must be aware of possible complications and how to manage them.

Indications

Central venous access is almost universal in intensive care patients. Indications include:

● Monitoring of CVP.
● Drug administration.
● Total parenteral nutrition.
● Fluid resuscitation.
● Insertion of temporary pacing wires.
● Insertion of pulmonary artery catheters.
● Dialysis.
● Lack of peripheral venous access.

Contraindications

These are relative but include severe coagulopathy, thrombocytopenia, and local sepsis.

You will need:

- Universal precautions. Sterile gown and gloves.
- Skin disinfectant.
- Sterile towels.
- 5-ml syringe of local anaesthetic.
- CVP line kit.
- Three-way taps.
- Heparinized saline to flush line.
- Suture.
- Dressing.
- ECG monitoring and defibrillator.

Central venous access may be achieved by a number of routes.

Internal jugular vein

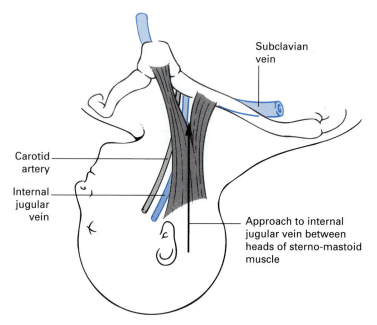

Fig. 13.1 Internal jugular vein.

Internal jugular vein cannulation is associated with a lower incidence of complications and higher incidence of correct line placement. It is especially appropriate for patients with severe coagulopathy or those patients with lung disease in whom pneumothorax may be disastrous. It may be best avoided in those patients with carotid artery disease or those with raised intracranial pressure because of the risks of carotid puncture and of impaired cerebral venous drainage.

The internal jugular vein runs from the jugular foramen at the base of the skull (immediately behind the ear) to its termination behind the posterior border of the sternoclavicular joint where it combines with the subclavian vein to become the brachiocephalic vein. Throughout its length it lies lateral, first to the internal and then common carotid arteries, within the carotid sheath, behind the sternomastoid muscle.

Many approaches to the internal jugular vein have been described. A typical approach is from the apex of the triangle formed by the two heads of the sternomastoid.

● Slightly extend the neck.
● Turn the head slightly to opposite side.
● Palpate the carotid artery at the level of the cricoid cartilage.
● To locate vein, introduce needle from the apex of the triangle at an angle of 30° and aim towards the ipsilateral nipple.

> **Warning!** It is a common mistake to assume the internal jugular vein is deep. Typically it is < 2 cm deep. It can easily be located with a short blue needle.

● Often when attempting to puncture the vein it collapses under the pressure of the needle and puncture is not recognized. The vessel may then be located by aspirating as the needle is slowly withdrawn. Blood will be aspirated as the needle tip passes back into the vein which refills once the pressure has been removed.

External jugular vein
The external jugular vein lies superficially in the neck, running down from the region of the angle of the jaw, across sternomastoid before passing deep to drain into the subclavian vein. It can be used to provide central venous access particularly in emergency situations when a simple large-bore cannula can be used for the administration of drugs and resuscitation fluids.

Subclavian vein (→ Fig. 13.2)
Subclavian vein cannulation is associated with a higher incidence of complications, particularly pneumothorax and a higher incidence of incorrect line placement than internal jugular cannulation. It is, however, more comfortable for the patient long-term and the site can more easily be kept clean.

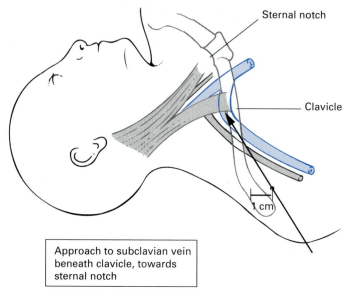

Sternal notch

Clavicle

1 cm

Approach to subclavian vein
beneath clavicle, towards
sternal notch

Fig. 13.2 Subclavian vein.

The subclavian vein begins at the apex of the axilla as a continuation of the axillary vein. It runs behind the posterior border of the clavicle and across the first rib to join the internal jugular vein, forming the brachiocephalic vein behind the sternoclavicular joint.

● Position patient supine (some people advocate placing a sandbag between the patient's shoulders blades. This allows the shoulders to drop back out of the way).
● Identify the junction of medial two-thirds and outer one-third of the clavicle.
● Introduce needle just beneath clavicle at this point, and aim towards clavicle until contact with bone is made.
● To locate vein redirect needle closely behind clavicle and towards the suprasternal notch.

Femoral vein
The femoral vein lies medial to the femoral artery immediately beneath the inguinal ligament. It is particularly useful for obtaining central access in small children and in patients with severe coagulopathy.

● Palpate femoral artery.
● To locate vein introduce needle 1 cm medial to femoral artery.

PROCEDURE

Central venous cannulae are of two types:

IV cannula over needle
Needle withdrawn and cannula left in situ through which a central venous line is inserted. Rarely used.

Catheter over guide wire
Seldinger wire through needle, needle withdrawn and central venous line passed over the wire. This type of central line is associated with a lower incidence of incorrect line placement and is the technique of choice.

● Where possible, position patient supine with 10–20° head down tilt. This distends the vein to aid location and helps prevent air embolism.
● Monitor ECG in case of arrhythmias (a defibrillator should be immediately available).
● Universal precautions.
● Use full aseptic technique, sterile gown and gloves.
● Prepare sterile field. (If planning internal jugular cannulation, it is a good idea to prepare the subclavian site at the same time and vica versa, in case of failure.)
● Prepare all equipment.
● Check wire passes through the needle freely. Attach three-way taps to all open ports of cannula. Flush the lumens with heparinized saline.
● Inject local anaesthetic to entry site. Do not forget to anaesthetize suture sites as well.
● Using a 10-ml syringe and needle enter central vein by chosen approach maintaining suction on the syringe at all times. If you appear to have missed the vein on the first pass pull back slowly whilst maintaining suction on the syringe. You often find you have gone through the vein and can find it on the way out.

Warning! Many people use a saline filled syringe to puncture the vessel. If you use a dry syringe to enter vein, it may be easier to determine whether the vessel entered is arterial or venous.

● Pass Seldinger wire through needle. This should pass freely and without any force into the vein. Watch for arrhythmias. Never pull the wire back through the needle once it has passed beyond the end of the bevel, it may shear off.
● Use scalpel (number 11 blade) to make a small nick in the skin. Hold the blade up and cut away from the wire.
● If provided pass dilator over the wire into the vein. Then remove it leaving wire in situ.

● Pass cannula over wire into vein. Make sure that before you push cannula forward the wire is visible at the proximal end. Hold on to the wire at all times, to prevent the wire being lost inside the patient!

● For an average adult patient the central venous cannula does not need to be inserted more than 12–15 cm. Check markings on the cannula. Most are 20 cm long and should not be inserted up to the hilt.

● Draw back blood, flush all the lumens of the line with heparinized saline and lock off the three-way taps. At this point the patient can be levelled.

● Suture the line into place using the anchorage devices provided and cover with a sterile dressing.

● Attach transducer and display wave form on monitor (see Fig. 13.3).

● Clear away and dispose of your sharps.

● CXR to verify position of line and check for complications including pneumothorax and haemothorax. Document the procedure in the patient's notes.

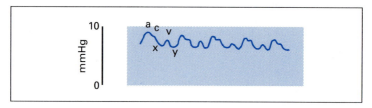

Fig. 13.3 CVP waveform.

Ultrasound guidance for vascular access

An increasing number of ICUs have a small portable ultrasound machine available to facilitate vascular access and other practical procedures. The use of these requires practice and you should use them on patients with normal anatomy and coagulation before moving on to more difficult cases.

Ultrasound allows:

● Direct visualization of the artery/vein and its associated structures.
● Identification of thrombosis, valve or anatomical abnormalities.
● Identification of best target vessel.
● First pass cannulation in the midline of a vessel directly avoiding other vital structures.

Arteries can be distinguished from veins by their round cross-section, non-compressibility and their pulsatility. Veins by contrast show respiratory fluctuation and are easily compressible.

In order to maintain sterility during vessel puncture put the ultrasound probe in a sterile plastic sheath.

COMMON PROBLEMS: CENTRAL VENOUS ACCESS

Cannot find the vein

Keep calm. Check your anatomical markings and try again. If unsuccessful do not persist with repeated passages of the needle in the hope of striking oil! Seek help.

 Warning! Do not procede immediately to the contralateral side: this increases the risk of complications, such as bilateral pneumothorax!

Needle in vein but cannot pass wire

Check needle position by drawing back on the syringe, good flow is essential. If OK, adjust the angle of incidence of the needle to the vein. Tip the patient further head down to further extend the vein. Try rotating the needle through 180° and draw back again. Remember the wire must pass easily without force. If this doesn't work repuncture the vein at a slightly different angle.

Is it arterial?

Occasionally, particularly if using a technique where the wire passes through the barrel of the syringe it is difficult to know whether you have hit the artery or the vein. In this case it is important to avoid passing a large central venous line into the vessel until you are sure. Consider the following:

● Connect a transducer directly to the needle in the vessel and look at the wave form.
● Pass the wire into the vessel and remove the needle. Pass a 18-gauge IV cannula over the wire into the vessel and remove the wire. Attach a transducer or manometer set directly to the cannula. When venous placement is confirmed pass wire back through IV cannula and continue as before.

Arterial puncture

● Needle only, then simply remove and press for 5 minutes.
● Large-bore cannula then action depends on circumstances. Usually can remove and press until bleeding stops. If severe coagulopathy leave in situ and give platelets and FFP before removing. Seek advice and consider the need for surgical exploration and removal under direct vision.

COMPLICATIONS

Complications of central venous cannulation depends in part on the route used, but include those in Table 13.2

TABLE 13.2 Complications of central venous cannulation

Early	Late
Arrhythmias	Infection
Vascular injury	Thrombosis
Pneumothorax	Embolization
Haemothorax	Erosion of vessels
Thoracic duct injury (Chylothorax)	
Pericardial tamponade	
Neural injury	

The management of pneumothorax depends upon the size of the pneumothorax and the patient's condition, particularly whether he/she is ventilated or not. A small pneumothorax in an unventilated patient with good gas exchange may be observed or aspirated using a small-bore cannula and syringe with three-way tap. Larger pneumothoraces, those that fail to resolve or those which cause any impairment of gas exchange and/or haemodynamics, require a formal chest drain. Small pleural caps of blood can be safely observed, but significant haemothorax should be formally drained as soon as possible. Once blood has clotted in the chest drainage is difficult. (See Chest drainage, p. 260.)

Bleeding around the puncture site can occasionally be a persistent problem. If pressure does not resolve this, use a suture (5/0 prolene) to tie a purse string around the puncture site. This usually stops the bleeding.

REMOVING AND CHANGING CENTRAL VENOUS LINES

Changing CVP lines

Line colonization with bacteria is common. Line related sepsis, defined as an unexplained episode of sepsis which resolves on removing the line occurs, in about 5–10% and is most commonly due to staphylococci.

It is reasonable, therefore, to change lines on a regular basis to prevent this. For example:

● All casualty and emergency resuscitation lines should be changed at 24 hours unless sited in the ICU with full aseptic technique.
● Other lines should be changed at 5 to 7 days depending on local policy (this is generally taken to include all central and arterial lines).

This is not a strict policy and will depend on the condition of the patient and the feasibility and ease of gaining alternative access. In general, lines should be placed at a clean site and if necessary the sites rotated to allow each access site to recover before being recannulated.

Changing lines over a wire

Occasionally a clean central venous line may need changing for an alternative. For example, a single lumen into a triple lumen or a central line into a pulmonary artery catheter. In this instance and particularly if access is difficult, lines may be changed over a wire. The technique is as for siting any central venous line.

- Cut sutures on the old line before scrubbing.
- Full aseptic technique.
- Clean and prep area.
- Pass wire down the central lumen of the old CVP line, and remove it, leaving wire in place. (Check the new wire is longer than the old CVP line.)
- Use the wire to site new line as required.

 Warning! The problem with this technique is keeping the new line sterile. Wear two pairs of gloves and discard the top pair when you have finished with the old line.

Removing central lines

To remove central lines ensure that all drugs and infusions have been stopped or relocated on to other lines. Lay patient down to reduce the risk of air embolism and remove the line smoothly applying pressure to the puncture site. Sit the patient up. Send the tip of the line in a dry specimen pot for culture.

LARGE BORE INTRODUCER SHEATHS

Introducer sheaths are available in a number of sizes for different applications. In adults 7.5 or 8.5 Fr. gauge are generally used. Smaller sheaths may be used for introducing specialized monitoring such as jugular bulb oximetry.

Indications

- Insertion of pulmonary artery catheter.
- Insertion of temporary pacing wire.
- Large line for volume resuscitation.

Procedure

Usually placed in the internal jugular or subclavian veins. The antecubital veins and femoral veins may be used, particularly in the presence of severe coagulopathy.

- Universal precautions.
- Full aseptic technique, sterile gown and gloves.
- Enter vein with needle, as for central venous line and pass Seldinger wire.
- Make small nick in the skin with a blade.
- Pass sheath mounted on the introducer/dilator over the wire into the vein.

Warning! The dilator is generally too long and does not need to be passed up to the hilt. Instead when the dilator has entered the vein over the wire, slide the sheath off the dilator without advancing the dilator any further.

● Remove wire and dilator. Draw back and flush with heparinized saline.
● When in situ and not in use the sheath port should be occluded with an obturator.
● Get CXR to check position and complications.

PULMONARY ARTERY CATHETERISATION

Indications for pulmonary artery catheterisation vary (See Table 13.3). Any condition where information derived will be useful in management, e.g. haemodynamically unstable patient who requires rationalization of fluid and inotrope therapy.

TABLE 13.3 Indications and contraindications for pulmonary artery catheterization

Indications	Contraindications
Shock	**Relative**
Sepsis	Severe coagulopathy
Valvular heart disease*	Unstable ventricular rhythm
Major trauma	Heart block
Heart failure	
Major surgery	**Absolute**
Extensive burns	Stenosis tricuspid or pulmonary valve
Pulmonary embolism	Mechanical tricuspid or pulmonary valve
Cor pulmonale/pulmonary hypertension	Temporary transvenous pacemaker (wire dislodgement)

* Relative indication: for example, in mitral stenosis and associated pulmonary hypertension the data obtained from pulmonary artery catheterization is often difficult to interpret, and there is an increased risk of pulmonary artery rupture.

You will need:

● Universal precautions. Sterile gown & gloves.
● Sterile towels.
● Skin cleaning solution.
● 5-ml syringe of local anaesthetic.

- Introducer sheath (see previous).
- Pulmonary artery catheter.
- Three-way taps.
- Heparinized saline to flush line.
- Transducer and monitor.
- ECG monitoring and defibrillator.

 Warning! Before attempting to insert a PA catheter ECG monitoring must be established and defibrillator must be immediately available because of the risks of arrhythmia.

Procedure

- Universal precautions.
- Full aseptic technique. Sterile gowns and gloves.
- Insert introducer sheath as previous.
- Flatten patient out before inserting PA catheter. (This reduces the pulmonary artery pressures and reduces the risk of pulmonary artery rupture.)
- Connect 3 three-way taps to the open ports, and flush lumens with heparinized saline.
- Connect 1.5-ml syringe to the balloon port and test the balloon. (Check the size of the balloon before starting.)
- Pass protective sleeve over PA catheter if provided.
- Pass the proximal end of the catheter to an assistant who can connect pressure transducer to the PA port (yellow) and flush the lumen. Then zero transducer and check the signal on the monitor. Need to display trace on the monitor (scale 0–75 mmHg) continuously.
- Calibrate fibreoptics if using a fibreoptic PA catheter.
- Insert PA catheter into introducer sheath and pass to 20 cm. Note normal CVP trace.
- Inflate balloon and advance catheter gently to right ventricle at approx. 30–40 cm. Advance further until the pulmonary artery is entered at approx. 40–50 cm.
- Advance catheter until pulmonary artery occlusion trace or wedge trace observed, approx. 20 cm from RV (approx. 50–60 cm total). Deflate balloon and see return of PA trace (see Fig. 13.4).

    Never:

- Never advance catheter with the balloon down.
- Never force the catheter.
- Never pass more than 20 cm of catheter without a change in the trace.
- Never overinflate the balloon.
- Never pull catheter back with balloon up.

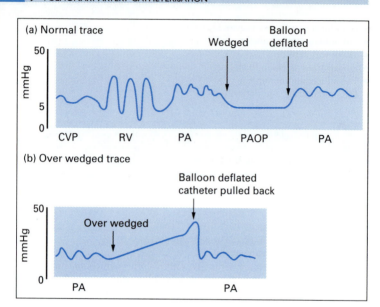

Fig. 13.4 Waveforms displayed while passing PA catheter.

COMMON PROBLEMS: PULMONARY ARTERY CATHETERIZATION

Catheter will not take the correct path

This may be due to a dilated RV or low cardiac output. Do not persist if unsuccessful.

- Remove completely, check direction of curvature of catheter and try again.
- To enter RV place patient head down and left side up.
- To enter PA place patient head up and supine.

Catheter is 'over wedged'

- Always watch the pressure trace when wedging the catheter. If pressure rises then catheter is 'over wedged'. (See Fig. 13.4.)
- The catheter is too distal within the PA. There is a risk of pulmonary artery rupture. Deflate balloon, pull catheter back and try again.

Catheter will not wedge

- This may be because the catheter is curled up within the PA. Do not pass more than 20 cm without a change in trace. Pull back and try again.

● In the presence of severe mitral regurgitation or pulmonary hypertension it may not be possible to obtain a satisfactory wedge trace and attempts may be associated with increased risk of PA rupture. Accept that catheter will not wedge and use pulmonary diastolic pressure instead of PA occlusion pressure.

CXR

● When catheter in position take CXR.
  – check position of catheter proximal (usually right) PA
  – exclude pneumothorax/haemothorax/widened mediastinum.

TABLE 13.4 Complications of pulmonary artery catheterization	
Central venous puncture	Any complications of central venous cannulation
Arrhythmia	Usually as pass through tricuspid valve and RV esp. if hypoxia, acidosis, hypokalaemia: Withdraw catheter and reposition.
Pulmonary infarction	Never leave balloon inflated
Pulmonary artery rupture	Avoid overinflation of balloon, watch trace and never inflate against resistance, pull back first
Infection	Careful aseptic technique and catheter care. Change after 72 hours
Knotting	Poor insertion technique. Do not insert more than 20 cm without a change in trace. Call for help. Do not attempt to pull back.

PA catheterisation is not without risk (see Table 13.4) and is certainly not a therapeutic manoeuvre. If patients are to benefit then regular collection and interpretation of haemodynamic and oxygen delivery variables together with the appropriate therapeutic response is required.

MEASURING PAOP

When measuring PAOP (Fig. 13.5) large variations in the wedge-pressure trace sometimes result from changes in mean thoracic pressure with respiration. It is, therefore, difficult to know where to position the cursor on the monitor in order to measure the wedge. The effects of mechanical or spontaneous ventilation can be discounted by positioning the cursor at that point which corresponds to end expiration.

MEASURING CARDIAC OUTPUT

There are now a number of methods of cardiac output measurement available, including oesophageal doppler ultrasound, and transthoracic impedance. The use of standard pulmonary artery catheters remains widespread.

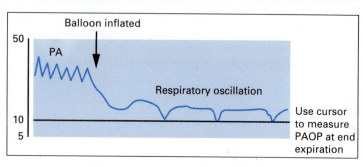

Fig. 13.5 Measuring PAOP.

Pulmonary artery catheters incorporate a thermistor near the tip to allow thermodilution measurement of cardiac output. A volume of cold 5% dextrose solution is injected through the central venous port of the PA catheter and the temperature change in the PA is detected by the thermistor. The degree and the rate of temperature change is used to calculate cardiac output.

● Ensure that the correct cables are connected between the monitor and the PA catheter (one to the distal thermistor and one to measure the temperature of the injectate).
● Check that the correct computation constant is entered into the monitor. This depends upon the volume and temperature of the injectate and also the type of catheter used. The correct computation constant is found on the packaging information of the PA catheter.

 Warning! It is best to use ice cold (4°C) 5% dextrose for the injectate. For convenience however, room temperature injectate is often used.

● Enter the patient's height and weight for calculation of body surface area (BSA).
● Set the computer to measure cardiac output, and when prompted inject 10 ml of 5% dextrose into the right atrial (CVP) lumen of the PA catheter. Time the injection at the end of inspiration and inject as rapidly as possible.
● Repeat the measurement. The individual cardiac output values obtained should not vary more than 5% from each other. Discard any inconsistent value and take the average reading for cardiac output.

Having measured the cardiac output and PA occlusion pressure a range of haemodynamic variables can be calculated. This is generally performed by the monitoring system. Normal values for these variables are shown in Table 13.5.

TABLE 13.5 Normal values for haemodynamic variables

Central venous pressure (CVP)	4–10 mmHg
Pulmonary artery occlusion pressure (PAOP)	5–15 mmHg
Cardiac output (CO)	4–6 l/min
Cardiac index (CI)	2.5–3.5 l/min/m²
Stroke volume (SV)	60–90 ml/beat
Stroke volume index (SVI)	33–47 ml/beat/m²
Systemic vascular resistance (SVR)	900–1200 dyne. s/cm⁵
Systemic vascular resistance index (SVRI)	1700–2400 dyne.s/cm⁵/m²
Pulmonary vascular resistance (PVR)	100–200 dyne. s/cm⁵
Pulmonary vascular resistance index (PVRI)	210–360 dyne.s/cm⁵/m²

In addition by measuring blood gases on blood drawn simultaneously from the pulmonary artery catheter and an arterial line, oxygen delivery and consumption variables may be calculated.

 Warning! Therapy is directed by the results of haemodynamic and oxygen delivery variables: It is important however, to treat the patient and not commence therapy on the basis of a single abnormal variable in a patient who is otherwise stable and maintaining adequate tissue and organ perfusion.

(See Optimizing haemodynamic status, p. 49) Oxygen delivery and consumption, p. 46.

PERICARDIAL ASPIRATION

Pericardial effusion and tamponade may be caused by a variety of medical conditions. The commonest cause overall is neoplasia, but in the ICU, chest trauma, including cardiothoracic surgery, and central venous access procedures are more likely causes. Although uncommon, the diagnosis should be considered in all patients who are at risk, and particularly in anyone who fails to respond to resuscitation.

The haemodynamic consequences of a pericardial effusion depend on the size and speed of accumulation. These include tachycardia, elevated central venous pressures, hypotension, pulsus paradoxus, and muffled heart sounds. None of these signs is specific and except in emergency circumstances pericardial aspiration should only be attempted after confirmatory echocardiogram.

Indications

- Cardiac tamponade.
- Large pericardial effusions.
- To obtain diagnostic pericardial fluid.

Contraindications

- Small loculated or posterior effusions (not causing haemodynamic compromise).

You will need:

- Universal precautions. Sterile gown and gloves.
- Skin cleaning solutions.
- Sterile towels.
- 10-ml syringe of local anaesthetic and needle.
- Pigtail catheter or 14 gauge single lumen central venous catheter (including syringe, needle and guide wire).
- Three-way tap.
- 50-ml syringe or vacuum drainage bottle.
- Suture.
- ECG monitoring, defibrillator and resuscitation equipment.

Procedure

- Explain procedure to patient. Place patient supine with 20° of head up tilt. Establish IV access if not already present and monitor ECG.
- Provide adequate sedation if necessary.
- Full aseptic technique. Sterile gowns and gloves.
- The point of needle insertion is immediately below and to the left of the xiphisternum, between the xiphisternum and left costal margin. Infiltrate the skin and subcutaneous tissue with local anaesthetic.
- Using 10-ml syringe advance needle at 45° to the patient, beneath the costal margin and towards the left shoulder aspirating continuously and observing the ECG.
- Fluid (straw coloured effusion or blood) is generally aspirated at a depth of 6–8 cm. Hold needle stationary and pass guide wire through needle into pericardial space.
- Remove needle, leaving guide wire in situ and then pass catheter over wire into pericardial space. Attach three-way tap.
- Use 50-ml syringe to aspirate pericardial effusion or attach to closed drainage system such as vacuum bottle.
- Suture drain in place.

Warning! Occasionally in emergency situation when aspirating presumed cardiac tamponade it is difficult to know whether blood aspirated is from the pericardial space or whether the ventricle has been punctured. Observe ECG throughout. If needle touches ventricle an injury pattern or arrhythmia will be obvious.

Complications

Performed carefully complications are few. These include pneumothorax, ventricular tachycardia, myocardial puncture and damage to the coronary arteries. A repeat CXR and echocardiogram should be performed after the procedure to confirm adequate placement and drainage and to identify any problems.

INTUBATION OF THE TRACHEA

This is the process whereby an endotracheal tube is passed orally or nasally into the trachea. This is covered at greater length in standard anaesthesia texts. However, there are some aspects of tracheal intubation of particular relevance to patients in intensive care.

 Warning! Do not attempt tracheal intubation without senior help if you are not experienced in the technique. In an emergency ventilate the patient with a bag and mask and await reinforcements!

Indications (Table 13.6)

These fall into two broad categories. Foremost is facilitation of artificial ventilation of the lungs and optimization of tissue oxygen delivery. The second is protection of the airway.

TABLE 13.6 Indications for tracheal intubation	
Facilitation of IPPV	**Airway protection**
Cardiopulmonary resuscitation	Risk of aspiration:
Anaesthesia and surgery	Obtunded conscious level
Respiratory failure	Neurological disease (bulbar problems)
Cardiac failure	
Multisystem organ failure	Airway obstruction
Major trauma including chest injury	Tumours
Brain injury	Head and neck trauma
	Croup, epiglottis
	Surgery
	Airway oedema

Patients requiring intubation in ICU differ from those in anaesthetic practice. They may already have an obtunded conscious level and limited physiological reserve, and so require minimal amounts of sedative agents. The judicious use of sedative drugs such as IV diazepam 5–10 mg may be all that is required. Anaesthetic induction agents in a low dose (e.g. propofol 1–2 mg/kg, etomidate 0.1–0.2 mg/kg) may be advantageous in blunting the pressor response in hypertensive patients and those with raised intracranial pressure. However over-zealous use of such agents in critically-ill patients may lead to cardiovascular collapse.

Muscle relaxant may be used to facilitate intubation. Only use a muscle relaxant if you are confident in airway skills. Suxamethonium 1–2 mg/kg is a short acting drug providing good intubating conditions and lasting only 3–4 minutes, so allows a margin of safety; it should be avoided in patients at risk of hyperkalaemia. Atracurium 0.4 mg/kg is a safe alternative but takes 2–3 minutes to achieve adequate relaxation for intubation and has a longer duration of action around 35 minutes.
(See Muscle Relaxants, p. 28.)

You will need:

- Skilled assistant.
- Self-inflating bag (Ambu or similar) and oxygen supply.
- Face mask.
- Suction and suction catheters.
- 2 laryngoscopes (check bulbs).
- Selection of endotracheal tubes.
- Syringe for cuff inflation and tape to tie tube.
- Gum-elastic bougie or rigid stilette.
- Resuscitation drugs – atropine, adrenaline, suxamethonium.

Procedure

- Preoxygenate the patient. Administer 100% oxygen by a tightly-fitted face mask for a period of 3–4 minutes prior to administering any drugs or attempting intubation, if possible. This will fill the functional residual capacity with oxygen, thereby increasing your safety margin.
- Check the head is in the 'sniffing the morning air' position (neck flexed, atlantoaxial joint extended, 1 firm pillow).
- If the patient has a full stomach, ask your assistant to apply cricoid pressure; if the neck is supported from behind and the cricoid firmly gripped, downward pressure prevents any passive regurgitation. If possible avoid inflating the lungs with the face mask and self-inflating bag until the tube is in place, as blowing air into the stomach may increase the risks of regurgitation.
- Any sedatives or relaxants may now be given.

Warning! If immediate intubation proves to be difficult or impracticable, do not persist with fruitless attempts. Ventilate the patient with 100% oxygen using bag and mask and call for help.

● Hold the laryngoscope in the left hand (size 3 or 4 Macintosh scopes are most commonly used). Slide the scope into the right of the mouth, sweeping the tongue into the groove in the blade, under it and to the left. As you advance the laryngoscope blade over the base of the tongue, the epiglottis pops into sight. With the blade between the epiglottis and the base of the tongue (vallecula), apply traction in the line of the laryngoscope handle, gently drawing the epiglottis forward and exposing the V-shaped glottis behind(Figs. 13.6 a&b).

● Pass the endotracheal tube between the vocal cords so that the cuff is just distal to them. Inflate the cuff while ventilating through the endotracheal tube with the self-inflating bag until any gas leak just disappears.

● Verify correct positioning of the tube by observation of chest movement, ausculation and if possible by capnography. Secure it, and attach to the ventilator via a suitable catheter mount. Recheck the tube position and chest movement.

● Final confirmation is by CXR. Check if the tube is too long, too short, endobronchial? Check for lobar collapse, pneumothorax, etc.

Complications

The commonest and immediately life threatening complication is oesophageal intubation. If in doubt, remove the tube, ventilate by face mask, and start again. Nasal intubation may provoke epistaxis or predispose to mucosal injury (e.g. submucosal positioning of the tube). In the longer term, nasal intubation may occlude the maxillary antrum and give rise to sinusitis. It is nevertheless better tolerated than oral intubation, particularly during weaning from ventilation. Long-term complications include erosion and stenosis of local tissues, particularly of the larynx and trachea. This may present as airway obstruction and stridor after extubation. See Miscellaneous problems: airway obstruction p. 216.)

Extubation

Before you consider extubation, the patient should be capable of breathing spontaneously with a satisfactory respiratory pattern and maintaining acceptable blood gases. They should have an appropriate conscious level and airway reflexes and not be requiring repeated airway suctioning. These precautions minimize the risks of laryngeal spasm and the need for early reintubation. (See Weaning from artificial ventilation, p. 87.)

● Check a suitable system for providing humidified oxygen by face mask is available, and you have everything necessary for reintubation.

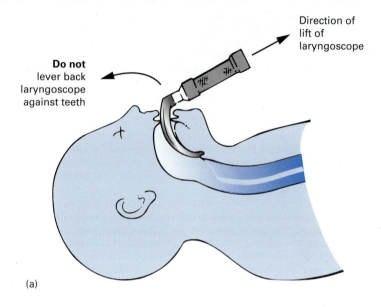

Direction of
lift of
laryngoscope

Do not
lever back
laryngoscope
against teeth

(a)

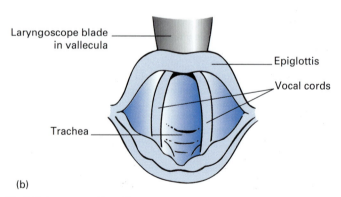

Laryngoscope blade
in vallecula

Epiglottis

Vocal cords

Trachea

(b)

Fig. 13.6 Laryngoscopy; View of larynx.

● Explain to the patient what you are going to do, then aspirate any secretions from the posterior pharynx.
● Insert a wide-bore suction catheter through the endotracheal tube. Deflate the cuff, and simultaneously aspirate through the suction catheter as you withdraw the endotracheal tube.

● Finally, fit the face mask and encourage the patient to cough out any further secretions.

TRACHEOSTOMY

There has been a resurgence of interest in the performance and use of tracheostomies in the ICU. Percutaneous tracheostomy kits enable tracheostomies to be safely and easily performed at the bedside. It is important to understand the procedure and the risks and benefits of tracheostomy. You should not perform these procedures without adequate training and supervision.

Indications

● Actual or impending airway obstruction. Tracheostomy should be considered early, before progressive swelling makes reintubation in the event of tube blockage or dislodgement potentially impossible.
● The need for prolonged IPPV (see below).
● Inability for the patients to protect or maintain their own airway in the longer term, e.g. severe brain injury, bulbar palsy.
● Aid to weaning.

Advantages

Tracheostomy has traditionally been considered after patients have been intubated for about 10–14 days. Many units are now performing tracheostomies earlier than this. Advantages include:

● Better tolerated than naso/oro-tracheal tubes, which allows significant reductions in muscle relaxants, sedative and analgesic drugs. This promotes return of GI tract function.
● Patients easily switched from IPPV/assist modes/CPAP/T piece without the need for extubation and reintubation.
● Easier clearance of tracheal secretions by suction.
● Speech is possible with cuff deflation.
● There may be a lower risk of airway problems after prolonged tracheostomy rather than prolonged translaryngeal intubation. Narrowing and scarring of the major airways is a potential risk in both situations.

Choices of tracheostomy

Tracheostomy may be safely performed through the cricothyroid membrane or in the subcricoid region. In the UK it is recommended that the tracheostomy stoma should be between the 2nd and 4th tracheal rings. At higher levels there may be an increased risk of laryngeal/tracheal stenosis, at lower level there is an increased risk of haemorrhage from major vessels in the thoracic inlet.

Increasingly the practice in ICUs is to perform percutaneous tracheostomies at the bedside to avoid the difficulties involved with moving patients to the operating theatre.

Percutaneous tracheostomy

Percutaneous tracheostomies can be performed without the use of specialized surgical instruments, specialized lighting or diathermy. The majority of patients are already intubated and ventilated and are given either an intravenous or volatile anaesthetic. This is supplemented by infiltration of the surgical area with 10 ml of local anaesthetic plus adrenaline which helps reduces skin edge bleeding. It is important to note that when the endotracheal tube is withdrawn to allow cannulation of the trachea, the airway may be lost if the tube is withdrawn too far. This may be prevented by passing a gum elastic bougie down the tube prior to withdrawal, or by using a laryngeal mask to maintain the airway rather than the endotracheal tube.

 Warning! This procedure requires a separate anaesthetist to manage the patient and airway and an operator to perform the tracheostomy. On no account should percutaneous tracheostomy be attempted by a single operator.

You will need:

● Anaesthetic assistance +/− anaesthetic machine.
● Nurse to help (not scrubbed).
● Universal precautions. Sterile gown and gloves.
● Skin disinfectant.
● Local anaesthetic (1% lignocaine + adrenaline) syringe and needle.
● 10 ml normal saline. Syringe.
● Basic surgical instruments (e.g., venous cut down set).
● Percutaneous tracheostomy kit.
● Appropriate size cuffed tracheostomy tubes (1 size smaller and larger than planned).
● Suture and securing tapes.

Procedure

Explain to the patient (and relatives) what you are going to do. Get written or verbal consent. Check the patient's coagulation status. Position the patient flat with the head and neck extended over a pillow.

Anaesthetist

● Ensure appropriate monitoring and anaesthetize patient with inhalational or intravenous technique as appropriate. Suction trachea and oropharynx. Ventilate with 100% oxygen throughout the procedure. When the operator is ready, withdraw the endotracheal tube under direct vision until cuff is visible at the laryngeal inlet. Care must be taken not to lose the airway. (Equipment must be available to reintubate the patient in case of difficulty.) Maintain ventilation until procedure is complete and then pass catheter mount to the operator.

Operator

● Position patient flat with the neck extended over a pillow.
● Clean skin.
● Palpate the cricothyroid membrane and sternal notch. Infiltrate skin with 1% lignocaine and adrenaline at a point midway between the two.
● Make a 2-cm superficial incision horizontally across the midline. This should only just break the skin.
● Use blunt forceps and a finger to dissect the pretracheal tissue until you can feel the tracheal rings and easily identify the position. If necessary tie off the anterior jugular veins which occasionally bleed.
● Ask the anaesthetist to withdraw the endotracheal tube until the tip is just within the larynx.
● Puncture the trachea with the introducer needle below the level of the first tracheal ring and in the midline. Using a saline filled syringe confirm the position of the needle by aspiration of air from the trachea. (A bronchoscope passed through the endotracheal tube can be used to confirm the correct position of the needle tip within the tracheal lumen.)
● Pass guide wire through the needle into the trachea.
● Remove the needle. Dilate the tract with the smallest short dilator and then introduce the protective sleeve over the guide wire. (This protects the guide wire from bending and is also notched to discourage you pushing the dilators too far.)
● Lubricate the dilators and dilate the tract using the sequential dilators to an appropriate size. (For adults this generally means using all the dilators in order to pass a size 8 tracheostomy tube.)
● Mount the tracheostomy tube on the appropriate size dilator for use as an introducer. Pass the introducer over the wire and slide tracheostomy tube off into the trachea. Remove the introducer and wire assembly.
● Suck out any blood from the trachea. Blood clot in the airway may produce total airway obstruction, or act as a ball valve allowing gas in but not out.
● Inflate the cuff and ventilate the patient through the tracheostomy.
● Correct placement of the tube is confirmed by the ability to pass a suction catheter easily, symmetrical chest expansion and bilateral breath sounds, maintenance of oxygenation, and capnography.
● Tie the tracheostomy in place using tracheostomy tapes. In addition it is advisable to place two stay sutures through the wings of the tracheostomy tube to prevent early accidental decannulation.
● A CXR should be performed to confirm position and exclude any complications.

COMMON PROBLEM: BLEEDING DURING PROCEDURE

Heavy bleeding from the wound may sometimes occur, particularly if an anterior jugular vein is damaged. If possible place a clip on the bleeding vessel and tie off. Otherwise pack the wound with gauze and wait, or if near the end of the procedure insert tracheostomy tube since this will often tamponade the bleeding. If bleeding does not stop, consider removing tracheostomy tube (reintubate the patient and pass endotracheal tube beyond stoma), pack the wound and seek surgical assistance.

COMMON PROBLEM: UNABLE TO VENTILATE PATIENT

This usually means that the tracheostomy tube has been misplaced. Do not persist as this may produce a tension pneumothorax! Remove the tracheostomy tube and reintubate the patient by the oral (nasal) route.

Complications (Table 13.7)

TABLE 13.7 Complications of tracheostomy	
Early	**Late**
Bleeding (may lead to total airway obstruction)	Tracheal stenosis
Pneumothorax	Tracheooesophageal fistula
Tube misplacement or dislodgement	Late haemorrhage from innominate vessels
Air emphysema	Infection round stoma site

Air emphysema is common but unless accompanied by a pneumothorax is unimportant and will resolve over time. Pneumothorax is generally the result of attempting to ventilate the patient through a misplaced tube, resulting in air tracking down into the mediastinum and pleural cavities.

Care of the patient with tracheostomy

Patients with tracheostomy tubes should receive adequate humidification of inspired gases to prevent drying and regular suction to removes secretions. Spare tracheostomy tubes of the same size and one size smaller should be kept at the bedside together with a pair of tracheal dilators.

Changing tracheostomy tubes

Tracheostomy tubes can be changed at any time if necessary, but is more difficult if the tract is not well established. Give patient 100% oxygen and position as for performing a tracheostomy. Pass a large-bore suction catheter (with the end cut off) or gum elastic bougie, through the old tracheostomy tube before removing it and use this as a guide to insert the new tube. Facilities for ventilating the patient with a bag and mask and for reintubation should be available in case of difficulty.

Decannulation

When the patient's condition has improved the question of when to remove the tracheostomy tube inevitably arises. Consideration should be given to the following:

● Respiratory effort.
● Volume of tracheal secretions and ability to cough spontaneously to clear them.
● Conscious level.
● Laryngeal competence and ability to swallow pharyngeal secretions.

There is no difficulty in a trial of decannulation, providing the tract is well formed (5–7 days after insertion). It is not routine practice to stitch up stomas, they are usually left to granulate on their own. A simple occlusive dressing should be applied over the stoma. If it is not possible to go for early decannulation, consideration should be given to changing a cuffed tracheostomy tube to non-cuffed fenestrated speaking tube. A number of such tubes exist with various valves to enable expiration to occur through the vocal cords to allow speech.

MINITRACHEOSTOMY

The term minitracheostomy has been coined to describe the insertion of a small-bore non-cuffed tube through the cricothyriod membrane (4 mm internal diameter). This technique has been used to aid secretion clearance after major surgery. The passage of suction catheters stimulates coughing and allows secretions to be aspirated. As a short-term measure these devices may help to prevent the need for naso/oro-tracheal intubation and assisted ventilation. The small size of the tube limits suction of viscid secretions and does not allow adequate ventilation or CPAP in the longer term. If a patient has very thick secretions, depression of conscious level, or is likely to shortly require ventilation then formal tracheostomy should be considered instead.

You will need:

● Universal precautions. Sterile gown and gloves.
● Skin disinfectant.
● Sterile drape.
● Syringe of local anaesthetic/needle/(10 ml of 2% lignocaine and adrenaline).
● Minitracheostomy kit (containing needle guide wire, dilator tube and tape).
● Suture.
● Dressing.

Procedure

Explain to the patient what you are going to do. Get written or verbal consent. Check the patient's coagulation status. Position the patient comfortably either sat up or laid down but with the head and neck extended over a pillow.

- Palpate anatomy to identify cricothyroid membrane and mark with pen.
- Clean neck with antiseptic solution.
- Infiltrate over cricothyroid membrane with 2–3 ml of local anaesthetic.
- Warn patient that you are going to make him cough and perform cricothyroid puncture with green 21 gauge needle. Aspirate air to confirm tracheal position of needle and rapidly inject 2 ml of lignocaine. Wait for coughing to subside.
- Perform superficial skin incision.
- Pass introducing needle into trachea and aspirate air.
- Pass guide wire through the needle and then remove the needle.
- Pass introducer over the guide wire and then slide minitracheostomy tube off the introducer. Remove introducer and guide wire together leaving minitracheostomy in place. Suction to remove any blood.
- Get CXR to verify the position.

Complications

The complications of minitracheostomy are the same as for formal tracheostomy. Misplacement and bleeding are particular problems.

BRONCHOSCOPY

Flexible fibreoptic bronchoscopy is a useful diagnostic and therapeutic tool in the ICU. In this situation it is usually performed on patients who have access to their airway via an endotracheal tube or tracheostomy.

Indications

- Removal of inspissated secretions (associated with areas of collapse on CXR).
- Retrieval of sputum samples for microbiology.
- Bronchial alveolar lavage (see below).
- Assessment of airway injury and burns.
- Biopsy of tumours and lung tissue.
- Assessment of endotracheal tube position.
- Fibreoptic intubation.

Contraindications

These are relative. Patients with high airway pressures, critical oxygenation and cardiovascular instability may not tolerate bronchoscopy.

Preparation

The bronchoscope should be sterilized before use according to hospital policy. This is generally by submersion in 2% glutaraldehyde for 20 minutes. This is a hazardous substance and you should wear gloves and goggles. The bronchoscope should then be rinsed off in sterile water and laid on a sterile green towel before use. Many hospitals now have automatic washers or involve CSSD.

Warning! When handling scope never allow it to bend or fold at acute angle as this will break the fibreoptic components.

You will need:

- Bronchoscope.
- Light source.
- Bowl of sterile water.
- Suction.
- Sputum traps.
- Sterile saline.
- Swivel connector with bronchoscopy port.
- Gown gloves and goggles.

Before commencing the procedure check that the size of the patient's endotracheal tube is adequate to allow bronchoscopy. Tubes smaller than size 8 may be significantly occluded by the bronchoscope, making ventilation and oxygenation of the patient difficult.

Procedure

- Attach the swivel connector to the patient's endotracheal or tracheostomy tube.
- Ventilate the patient on 100% oxygen prior to and during the bronchoscopy.
- Adequately sedate the patient and then give a small dose of muscle relaxant (such as atracurium) to prevent the patient biting or coughing on the bronchoscope. It is sensible to have an assistant to look after patient sedation and ventilation whilst you perform the bronchoscopy.
- Bronchoscopy should be a clean procedure to avoid contaminating the patient's airway.
- Lubricate scope with a small amount of lubricant jelly. Avoid getting it over the lens. Pass bronchoscope through the bung on the swivel connector and into the endotracheal or tracheostomy tube. Continue forward under direct vision.

 Warning! Use of the bronchoscope clearly requires a knowledge of the endoscopic anatomy of the bronchial tree (see Fig. 13.7).

- Pass the scope forward to the carina. Then explore each side of the bronchial tree in turn. Identify and enter each lobar and segmental bronchus. Take note of any abnormal anatomy and remove any secretions.

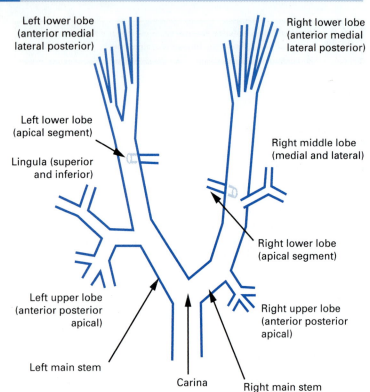

Fig. 13.7 Anatomy of bronchial tree.

● If thick secretions are present that cannot be sucked up the scope try instilling 10–20 ml of sterile saline down the suction port of the bronchoscope. This may help to loosen them. Large plugs and blood clots may be dragged out on the end of the scope.

● To obtain microbiology specimens place a sputum trap in between the bronchoscope and the wall suction. Use a separate trap for each side. Be careful to keep the sputum trap upright to prevent the secretions disappearing down the suction tubing. Also remove sputum traps before removing scope from the patient to prevent specimens being contaminated with upper airway flora.

● Bronchial biopsy should not be performed by trainees in intensive care.

● Following bronchoscopy perform a CXR to exclude pneumothorax and look for improvement in lung expansion where large sputum plugs have been removed.

Warning! After bronchoscopy it is your responsibility to clean the bronchoscope. Suck a large bowl of water through the suction channel and then pass a suction channel brush down the scope to remove any particulate matter. Dismantle the suction port valves and scrub these with a brush and soapy water. Then wash the whole scope with soapy water. Finally the scope should be sterilized according to your hospital policy.

BRONCHIAL ALVEOLAR LAVAGE (BAL)

(BAL) is a technique for obtaining microbiology specimens from low in the respiratory tree, avoiding contamination of samples with upper respiratory tract flora. It may be performed during bronchoscopy or using specially designed BAL catheters.

Indications
BAL may be used to obtain specimens in any patient with pneumonia. It is of particular value in investigating pneumonia in the immunocompromised patient. In addition to conventional pathogens such as *Streptococcus pneumoniae* and *Haemophillus influenzae* other likely pathogens in these patients are *Pneumocystis carinii*, either alone or with a copathogen, mycobacterium species including tuberculosis, cytomegalovirus and fungi.

Discuss the clinical situation with a microbiologist before performing the BAL. They will advise on appropriate specimens and tests.

BAL during bronchoscopy
This has the advantage that the operator can be highly selective in the area for lavage in the case of localized disease. It is, however, more invasive and operator dependant.

● During bronchoscopy (see previous) the bronchoscope is passed into a subsegmental bronchus until it wedges.
● Up to 100 ml of saline is instilled down the suction channel.
● This is then aspirated and collected into a series of sputum traps.

Warning! Not all the saline instilled will be aspirated back. This does not matter provided that a reasonable specimen is obtained.

BAL using catheter
BAL catheters consist of a protective outer sleeve and an inner suction catheter. The suction catheter can be connected via a three-way tap to suction and a syringe for instilling saline. This should be a clean procedure and you should wear apron, gloves and goggles.

- Preoxygenate the patient with 100% oxygen.
- Pass catheter, with inner tube protected, into airway, beyond the endotracheal tube.
- Advance the inner protected suction catheter forwards until it meets resistance. Do not use undue force.
- Perform BAL according to local protocol. Generally 80–100 ml of saline are instilled down the suction catheter, and then aspirated into 2 or 3 sputum traps. Not all the saline may be aspirated. This does not matter.
- Withdraw inner suction catheter into protective sleeve before removing from patient.

Having performed a BAL, telephone the laboratory and then send samples immediately with full diagnostic information and appropriate requests.

Investigations following BAL

Urgent Gram and ZN stain
Microscopy culture & sensitivity incl. TB (AAFB)
Differential cell count
Fungi
Viruses
Legionella immune fluorescent antibody test
Pneumocystis carinii

CHEST DRAINAGE

Warning! The emergency treatment of life threatening tension pneumothorax is large-bore needle decompression. The diagnosis is made on clinical grounds without CXR. A 14-gauge cannula is inserted into the pleural cavity immediately above the second rib in the midclavicular line. This should be followed by formal chest drainage.

Indications
Chest drains are indicated for the drainage of air (pneumothorax), blood (haemothorax), fluid (pleural effusion), pus (empyema), and lymph (chylothorax) from the pleural cavity.

For small focal collections, a pigtail catheter may be inserted under ultrasound or other radiological control.

Site of drain

This is partly dictated by the position of the collection clinically and radiographically. In the case of long standing collections, which may be loculated, ultrasound guidance may be helpful. In most cases the drain should be sited in the 5th intercostal space, just anterior to the midaxillary line, and can be directed cephalad for air and caudally for fluid or blood. All drains should be placed immediately above the rib to avoid damage to the neurovascular bundle which lies underneath.

 Warning! 2nd Intercostal space midclavicular line. This site is associated with risk of injury to breast tissue in the female and may result in significant cosmetic scarring. It should be avoided.

You will need:

- Universal precautions sterile gown and gloves.
- Skin disinfectant.
- Sterile drape.
- 10 ml syringe local anaesthetic and needles (lignocaine 2%).
- Basic instruments: scalpel, blade, large arterial clamps.
- Chest drain.
- Strong silk sutures, adhesive strapping and dressings.
- Underwater seal, low-pressure vacuum (wall vacuum or pump).

Procedure

- Explain procedure to patient.
- Position patient (supine with arm lifted, a pillow behind back).
- Prepare a sterile field.
- Infiltrate superficial structures down to rib with local anaesthetic.
- Make a 4-cm incision.
- Palpate through skin incision and perform blunt dissection down to rib and through pleura.
- Push finger into pleural cavity and sweep around to ensure no viscera are adjacent.
- Insert drain and direct into appropriate position.

 Warning! Trocars should not be used to insert drains. These are sharp and may cause injury to underlying viscera.

- Connect to underwater drain and confirm position by drainage of collection and respiratory swing.

- Secure drain in position with suture. Purse string sutures result in very unsightly scarring when chest drains are removed and are best avoided. Use mattress sutures to close the skin edges and a simple tie to hold in the drain.
- Get CXR to confirm position.

Warning! Chest drains should not be clamped. If moving a patient, simply keep the underwater bottle below the level of the chest. Clamping drains may produce a tension pneumothorax.

COMMON PROBLEM: LUNG WILL NOT EXPAND

Reassess diagnosis and position of tube. Is tube swinging? Is the effusion loculated?

- Consider low-pressure high-volume suction (wall suction or pump 10–20 mmHg).
- Increase tidal volume or add 10 cm of PEEP.
- Consider need for surgical referral (see below).

COMMON PROBLEM: PERSISTENT AIR LEAK

Check the drain and reposition if necessary (it may have come out of the chest and be sucking room air). If air leak persists attempt to minimize airway pressures.

- In trauma patients, consider bronchoscopy to exclude airway rupture.
- Wean patient onto spontaneous breathing modes if appropriate.
- If ventilated, ensure adequate sedation analgesia and muscle relaxation.
- Use pressure controlled ventilation and reduce PEEP.
- Accept a degree of hypercapnia, e.g. $Pa\mathrm{CO_2}$ 8 kPa.
- Consider high frequency jet ventilation.

The combination of persistent air leak and non-compliant lungs (e.g. ARDS) may make adequate ventilation and gas exchange impossible. Seek urgent thoracic surgical opinion.

Indications for surgical opinion/thoracotomy
Collection not fully drained or lung not fully re-expanded
Massive air leak (bronchopleural fistula/ruptured bronchus)
Continued bleeding
Presence/suspected presence other intrathoracic injuries

Removing chest drains

Chest drains can be removed when they are no longer needed. In practice, this means that if the clinical and CXR findings that required a chest drain have resolved, and the drain is no longer bubbling or draining fluid, it can be removed.

● There is no need to clamp drains before removal.
● Clean the site with antiseptic solution. Cut the retaining suture, remove the drain and occlude by pressing.
● Close the wound with a suture. If this is already in situ it can be tied as the drain is removed to reduce any air entrainment. (Avoid purse strings as above.)
● Obtain a CXR.

PASSING A NASOGASTRIC TUBE

All patients in the ICU who require ventilation require a nasogastric tube to ensure gastric drainage and early enteral feeding (see Table 13.8).

TABLE 13.8 Indications and contraindications for nasogastric intubation	
Indications	**Contraindications**
To deflate the stomach after ventilation with a bag and mask	Base of skull fracture (use oral gastric tube)
To aspirate gastric contents which might otherwise reflux and soil the airway	Recent gastric or oesophageal surgery (call surgeon)
To provide a route for enteral feeding and drugs	Oesophageal varices (relative contraindication)
	Severe coagulopathy (consider oral route to avoid nose bleed)

You will need:

● Gloves and mask.
● NG tube.
● Lubricating jelly.
● Laryngoscope.
● Magill forceps.

Procedure

● Explain to the patient what you are going to do, even if he/she is apparently unconscious. Position the patient supine with head neutral.
● Lubricate the NG tube and keeping alignment with the long axis of the patient introduce through the nose. Do not force. If resistance is met try the other side.
● If the patient is co-operative ask them to swallow the tip of the tube when he/she feels it in the back of the throat. In unconscious patients the tube may pass directly into the oesophagus but often coils up in the mouth.
● In this case use a laryngoscope to examine the pharynx and pass the tube manually into the oesophagus using a pair of Magill forceps. (Be careful not to traumatize the uvula and pharyngeal mucosa.)

● Confirm the position of the NG tube in the stomach by aspiration of gastric contents (turns litmus paper red), auscultation (gurgling when air blown into tube) or by CXR.

● Secure the NG tube in position with adhesive tape.

GASTRIC TONOMETRY

This is a method of estimating gastric mucosal pH. It is useful because it reflects splanchnic blood flow changes which may be important in the development of SIRS and multiple organ failure. (See Gastrointestinal tract, p.108 and sepsis, p. 200.)

Principle

A specially designed NG tube with a silicon balloon on the distal end is passed into the stomach. The balloon is filled with saline and carbondioxide produced from the cells of the gastric mucosa can diffuse into this, while hydrogen ions which are free within the lumen of the stomach cannot.

The saline in the balloon, therefore, equilibrates with intragastric P_{CO_2} which in turn reflects the mucosal intracellular P_{CO_2}. If the arterial bicarbonate concentration is known (and this is assumed to reflect intracellular bicarbonate concentration) then the Henderson–Hasselbalch equation can be used to estimate the intracellular pH (pHi).

Procedure

● Prior to insertion all air must be aspirated from the balloon. A syringe of saline is attached to the three-way tap and with the catheter tip angled downward, 4 ml of saline is instilled into the balloon. This is then aspirated and the process repeated until all air bubbles are cleared from the tonometry lumen.

● With the balloon collapsed the tonometry catheter is passed into the stomach. Position can be confirmed by CXR.

● A 5-ml syringe of saline is attached to the three-way tap and 2.5 ml is irrigated through the side port. The remaining 2.5 ml is instilled into the balloon. The tap is closed and the time recorded.

● An equilibration time of 30–90 min is allowed and the time again recorded.

● The first 1 ml of the saline is aspirated from the balloon and then discarded through the side port of the three-way tap (without disconnecting the syringe). The remaining 1.5 ml is then aspirated until the balloon is empty.

● The sample is capped and transported on ice to the blood gas machine for immediate analysis. At the same time an arterial sample is also taken for bicarbonate measurement.

● The P_{CO_2} measured from the saline is corrected to allow for incomplete equilibration between the gastric luminal CO_2 and the saline. This corrected P_{CO_2} is the steady state measurement $P_{CO_2}ss$. (A table of correction factors is supplied with the tonometer.)

● pHi is then calculated from the Henderson–Hasselbalch equation.

$$pHi = 6.1 + \log \frac{(HCO_3-)}{P\text{CO}_2\text{ss} \times 0.03} \qquad P\text{CO}_2\text{ss in mmHg}$$

Alternatively a slide rule is provided with the tonometer which calculates $P\text{CO}_2\text{ss}$ and pHi directly from measured $P\text{CO}_2$ and arterial bicarbonate.

New automated devices for measuring pHi are now being produced. These avoid the complicated procedure described above which limits the usefulness of the conventional gastric tonometer.

Intramucosal pHi values below 7.3 imply inadequate splanchnic perfusion and oxygen delivery, and have been associated with adverse outcomes.

SENGSTAKEN–BLAKEMORE TUBE

A number of tubes have been designed to apply pressure to oesophageal varices in order to compress the vessels and reduce bleeding, whilst the patient is resuscitated and definitive treatment carried out. The Sengstaken – Blakemore tube has three lumens. Two are used to inflate balloons, one in the stomach and the other in the oesophagus whilst the third is used to aspirate gastric contents.

You will need:

● Universal precautions.
● Suction apparatus.
● Sengstaken – Blakemore tube (usually kept in a fridge).
● 500 ml saline.
● 50 ml syringe.
● Traction (string and 500 ml bag of fluid).

Procedure

● Read instructions for specific device you are using!
● Explain to the patient what you are going to do.
● Position the patient comfortably. Left lateral is best if the patient is vomiting.
● Check the patency of the tube lumens and integrity of the balloons.
● Pass the tube orally into the oesophagus and down into the stomach.
(Local anaesthetic spray to the pharynx may make this more tolerable in the awake patient.) Insert the tube to at least 30 cm.
● Inflate the gastric balloon with 250 ml of saline. You should not feel any resistance.
● Pull the tube backwards gently until resistance is felt as the gastric balloon meets the gastrooesophageal junction.
● Inflate the oesophageal balloon with air or saline (approximately 100 ml). The pressure in the oesophageal balloon can be measured using a sphygmomanometer and should be 25–35 mmHg. Chest pain, respiratory difficulty and cardiac arrhythmias may occur during inflation of the balloon.

● Apply traction to the tube by tying a piece of string to the end and suspending a 500-ml bag of fluid over a fulcrum. Traction should be released at regular intervals to prevent pressure necrosis of the gastrooesophageal junction.

● The position of the tube should be checked by CXR. The point where the tube exits the mouth should be marked in order to detect subsequent migration. Check the pressure in the oesophageal balloon regularly.

Removing the tube

After 24 hours the traction should be removed and the oesophageal balloon deflated to assess for bleeding. If bleeding recurs the balloon can be reinflated for a further period of 24 hours, however, the need for surgery becomes increasingly likely. If there is no bleeding the tube is generally left in situ deflated for 24 hours in case bleeding recurs. After this time the tube can be removed.

TRANSPORTING PATIENTS

Interhospital transport is a specialist area. However, most junior doctors involved in intensive care will have to perform such a transfer at some stage.

The standard of care for interhospital transfers should be the same as that provided within an ICU. Before transporting the patient, it is important that the patient is fully resuscitated. If there is any doubt regarding the adequacy of resuscitation, this should be addressed before transfer. You should also take with you any drugs, resuscitation equipment, and syringe pumps that you are likely to need during the transfer. Check that the ambulance has a source of suction.

● Full monitoring should be employed. This includes blood pressure monitoring (preferably invasive) ECG, oxygen saturation, and end-tidal CO_2 where available.

● Ensure that the airway is secure, this invariably means endotracheal intubation.

● Ensure adequate supplies of oxygen to complete the transfer. In case the supply fails, an alternative means of ventilating the patient should be available. This should be a self-inflating bag, rather than an anaesthetic breathing circuit.

● Ensure adequate intravenous access. This usually means at least two intravenous cannulae.

The staff undertaking the transfer should be adequately trained; you should take with you an intensive care nurse or an ODA. The transfer should be fully documented, including a record of pulse, blood pressure, ventilation and other vital signs. Departure and arrival times should be notified to the receiving hospital sufficiently in advance that suitable preparation can be made.

CHAPTER 14

APPENDIX DRUG INFORMATION

NB The following notes and drug doses are for guidance only, based on 70-kg adult. Exact doses will depend upon the requirement and the patient's condition. For further information seek advice from senior or pharmacist, or refer to the BNF.

*For notes on anaesthetic and sedative drugs and muscle relaxants, see relevant sections.

Drug	Method of Administration	Notes
N-Acetylcysteine	Continuous infusion 100 mg/kg in 250–1000 ml 5% dex. over 16 h	
Adrenaline	5 mg in 50 ml 5% dex. 0.1–1 µg/kg/min	Increase concentration and dose according to response
Aminophylline	Loading dose 5 mg/kg over 20 min Maintenance 0.5–0.8 mg/kg/h	Omit loading if already receiving theophyllines. Increase dose in smokers. Reduce dose if receiving concurrent erythromycin or cimetidine. Check levels
Amiodarone	300 mg in 250 ml 5% dex. over 1 h followed 900 mg in 500 ml over 24 h then 1200 mg in 500 ml over 24 h.	Half dose after 48 h
Calcium Gluconate	10 ml 10% calcium gluconate slow IV bolus, or infusion in 5% dex.	Precipitates with sulphates, bicarbonates and phosphates
Digoxin	Loading dose 0.5–1 mg in 50 ml 5% dex. over 30 min Maintenance 62.5–250 µg over 30 min daily	Check levels
Dobutamine	250 mg/50 ml 5% dex. 0–20 µg/kg/min	Increase concentration and dose according to response
Dopamine	200 mg/50 ml 5% dex. 2.5–5 µg/kg/min renal dose	
Dopexamine	50 mg/50 ml 5% dex. 0–5 µg/kg/min	
Enoximone	100 mg/40 ml 0.9% saline loading up to 90 µg/kg/min maintenance 5–20 µg/kg/min	Beware hypotension. Loading dose often best avoided. Max 24 h 24 mg/kg

Drug	Method of Administration	Notes
GTN	50 mg/50 ml (neat) 0–0.5 µg/kg/min	
Heparin	5000 units IV loading dose 500–2000 units/hour IV according to indication	Monitor APTT
Hydralazine	5–10 mg IV bolus repeated as necessary. If required continuous infusion 50 mg/500 ml 0.9% saline 0.05–0.3 mg/min	
Insulin	50 units in 50 ml 0.9% saline continuous infusion as required	Monitor blood sugar
Isoprenaline	10 mg/100 ml 5% dex. 0–0.5 µg/kg/min	
Labetalol	100 mg/20 ml (neat) IV bolus 5–20 mg infusion start at 15 mg/h double every 30 min to a maximum of 160 mg/h according to response	
Lignocaine	IV bolus 1 mg/kg (100 mg) infusion 1 g/500 ml 5% dex. 2–4 mg/min	
Noradrenaline	4 mg/50 ml 5% dex. 0.1–0.5 µg/kg/min	Increase concentration and dose according to response
Phenylephrine	100 mg in 100 ml 5% dex. 0–10 µg/kg/min	
Potassium chloride	10–20 mmol/20–50 ml 0.9% saline over 30 min	Give via central line. Monitor ECG
Phenytoin	15 mg/kg loading slow IV injection Maintenance 3–5 mg/kg daily	Do not exceed 50 mg/min. Monitor levels
Prostacycline	250 µg in 50 ml 0.9% saline 5–10 ng/kg/min	
Salbutamol	200–300 µg IV bolus repeated if necessary, infusion 5 mg/500 ml 5% dex. 5–20µg/min	
Streptokinase	1.5 mega units in 0.9% saline over 60 min	

DRUG LEVELS

The following drugs require monitoring of plasma levels either to ensure that therapeutic levels are obtained or to avoid potential toxicity.

Drug	When to take sample	Desired levels
Cyclosporin	Predose (trough)	100–250 ng/ml
Digoxin	> 6 h postdose	1–2.6 nmol/l
Gentamicin	Predose (trough)	< 2 mg/l
	1 h postdose	5–10 mg/l
Phenytoin	> 4 h postdose	10–20 mg/l
Tacrolimus	Predose (trough)	5–20 ng/ml
Teicoplanin	Predose (trough)	10–15 mg/l
	1 h postdose	up to 40 mg/l
Theophylline	2 h postdose	10–20 mg/l
	(unless on continuous infusion)	
Tobramycin	Predose (trough)	< 2 mg/l
	1 h postdose	5–10 mg/l
Vancomycin	Predose (trough)	5–10 mg/l
	2 h post dose	18–26 mg/l

In general if:

● Trough level high, omit until a random level is within the desired range and then increase the period between doses.
● Peak level high, reduce the dose.

INDEX